COMPACT *Research*

Digestive Disorders

Peggy J. Parks

Diseases and Disorders

ReferencePoint Press®

San Diego, CA

ReferencePoint Press®

For more information, contact:
ReferencePoint Press, Inc.
PO Box 27779
San Diego, CA 92198
www.ReferencePointPress.com

Picture credits:
Cover credit: Dreamstime and iStockphoto.com
Maury Aaseng: 31–33, 45–47, 59–61, 74–76
Science Photo Library: 11, 13

LIBRARY OF CONGRESS CATALOGING-IN-PUBLICATION DATA

Parks, Peggy J., 1951–
Digestive disorders / by Peggy J. Parks.
pages cm. -- (Compact research series)
Audience: Grade 9 to 12.
Includes bibliographical references and index.
ISBN 978-1-60152-514-7 (hardback) -- ISBN 1-60152-514-1 (hardback)
1. Digestive organs--Diseases--Juvenile literature. 2. Gastrointestinal system--Diseases--Juvenile literature. I. Title.
RC801.P345 2014
616.3--dc23

2012051710

Contents

Foreword

“Where is the knowledge we have lost in information?”

—T.S. Eliot, “The Rock.”

As modern civilization continues to evolve, its ability to create, store, distribute, and access information expands exponentially. The explosion of information from all media continues to increase at a phenomenal rate. By 2020 some experts predict the worldwide information base will double every seventy-three days. While access to diverse sources of information and perspectives is paramount to any democratic society, information alone cannot help people gain knowledge and understanding. Information must be organized and presented clearly and succinctly in order to be understood. The challenge in the digital age becomes not the creation of information, but how best to sort, organize, enhance, and present information.

ReferencePoint Press developed the *Compact Research* series with this challenge of the information age in mind. More than any other subject area today, researching current issues can yield vast, diverse, and unqualified information that can be intimidating and overwhelming for even the most advanced and motivated researcher. The *Compact Research* series offers a compact, relevant, intelligent, and conveniently organized collection of information covering a variety of current topics ranging from illegal immigration and deforestation to diseases such as anorexia and meningitis.

The series focuses on three types of information: objective single-author narratives, opinion-based primary source quotations, and facts and statistics. The clearly written objective narratives provide context and reliable background information. Primary source quotes are carefully selected and cited, exposing the reader to differing points of view, and facts and statistics sections aid the reader in evaluating perspectives. Presenting these key types of information creates a richer, more balanced learning experience.

For better understanding and convenience, the series enhances information by organizing it into narrower topics and adding design features that make it easy for a reader to identify desired content. For example, in *Compact Research: Illegal Immigration*, a chapter covering the economic impact of illegal immigration has an objective narrative explaining the various ways the economy is impacted, a balanced section of numerous primary source quotes on the topic, followed by facts and full-color illustrations to encourage evaluation of contrasting perspectives.

The ancient Roman philosopher Lucius Annaeus Seneca wrote, "It is quality rather than quantity that matters." More than just a collection of content, the *Compact Research* series is simply committed to creating, finding, organizing, and presenting the most relevant and appropriate amount of information on a current topic in a user-friendly style that invites, intrigues, and fosters understanding.

Digestive Disorders at a Glance

Digestive Disorders Defined

Any conditions that affect the human digestive system are known as digestive disorders.

A Wide Variety

Scientists have identified a wide variety of digestive disorders that range in severity from mild heartburn or constipation to life-threatening bowel diseases.

Prevalence

The National Institute of Diabetes and Digestive and Kidney Diseases (NIDDK) estimates that up to 70 million people in the United States suffer from digestive disorders.

Causes

The exact cause of most digestive disorders is unknown, although scientists believe that genetic and environmental factors are involved.

Effects

Depending on their type and severity, digestive disorders can severely affect a sufferer's quality of life; young people can have an especially difficult time coping with these disorders.

Diagnosis

Diagnosing a digestive disorder involves a physical examination, medical history, and a variety of different tests, depending on the patient's symptoms and what illness is suspected.

Prevention Strategies

Digestive disorders cannot typically be prevented, although many can be successfully managed through a more nutritious diet and healthier lifestyle.

Treatment

Many digestive disorders can be successfully treated if sufferers seek medical attention early; treatment plans are developed based on which disorder is involved and the individual needs of the patient.

Overview

"Digestive diseases are among the leading causes of doctor visits, hospitalizations, and disability in the U.S. each year."

The National Institute of Diabetes and Digestive and Kidney Diseases, which conducts and supports medical research and research training to improve people's health and quality of life.

"Many children have tummy aches and other digestive problems, and they usually are not serious. But sometimes these common childhood ailments can be the sign of something that needs medical attention."

University of Maryland Medical Center, a teaching hospital located in Baltimore that provides a full range of health care to people throughout Maryland and the mid-Atlantic region.

Alexander Noyes is a professional drummer who has Crohn's disease, a digestive disorder characterized by severe abdominal pain and rectal bleeding. Diagnosed when he was eighteen years old, Noyes says that at first he thought that his condition was not a big deal. He was so unconcerned, in fact, that he threw away the medications prescribed by his doctor. "I think some part of you is in denial at that point, especially at that age," he says. "You kind of have a feeling of invincibility [as if you are] bigger than the disease."[1] As Noyes's health continued to deteriorate, it became painfully obvious that he was *not* "bigger" than his disease. At the time, he was a member of the Jonas Brothers and went on tour with the band. There were nights when it took every bit of strength he had to keep going, and sometimes he was in the bathroom throwing up just minutes before going onstage to perform.

Finally, after a year and a half of a grueling touring schedule, Noyes could no longer deny the severity of his disease. He was feeling sick all the time and had undergone so many flare-ups that thick scar tissue had formed in his small intestine, which necessitated corrective surgery. The operation was performed in December 2007, and Noyes has had no flare-ups since. He has a renewed commitment to take care of his health by watching his diet, visiting his doctors on a regular basis, and taking his medication faithfully. Through his painful ordeal he learned the importance of proper management of his illness, and he also learned something else—the value of a sense of humor when times get really tough. "If you can't laugh at the situation," he says, "it can become overwhelming."[2]

How Digestion Works

Crohn's disease is one of numerous disorders that affect the digestive system, which scientists, physicians, and other health-care professionals commonly refer to as the "gut." It consists of the digestive tract (also known as the alimentary canal or gastrointestinal tract) and the abdominal organs that help the body break down and absorb food; namely, the liver and pancreas. The digestive tract is composed of a series of hollow organs joined in a long, twisting tube. It includes the mouth; the esophagus, which is a muscular tube that connects the throat above to the stomach below; the stomach itself; the small intestine (or small bowel); the large intestine (the colon or large bowel); the rectum; and the anus.

> **From the time food is chewed and swallowed, it begins to move through the digestive system in a meticulously coordinated process.**

During digestion, food is broken down into nutrients that can be used as fuel by the body's cells. Georgia College and State University distinguished biology professor Kenneth S. Saladin writes: "The digestive system is essentially a disassembly line—its primary purpose is to break nutrients down into forms that can be used by the body and to absorb them so they can be distributed to the tissues."[3] From the time food is chewed and swallowed, it begins to move through the digestive system in a meticulously coordinated process. It travels down the throat and into the esophagus where a wave of muscle contractions (known as peristalsis) forces it downward. The lower esophageal sphincter (LES), which is a small, circular muscle at the bottom of the esophagus, relaxes and opens briefly to allow the food to pass into the stomach. Then like a valve, the muscle squeezes shut to keep the food from flowing back up into the esophagus.

> **“Through years of research, scientists have identified a wide variety of digestive disorders. These range in severity from conditions that are uncomfortable but not particularly serious to those that can be life threatening.”**

The stomach muscles begin to churn and mix the food with digestive juices consisting of hydrochloric acid and enzymes. Kenneth Koch, a gastroenterologist (digestive disease specialist) from Winston-Salem, North Carolina, describes this part of the digestive process: “The stomach is an expandable receiving chamber. You can think of it as a powerful yet gentle mill that grinds your food down to millions of tiny pieces for hours after you eat even though you don't feel a thing.”[4] This time the “mill” changes food into a paste-like substance known as chyme. Another sphincter muscle, the pyloric sphincter, then relaxes and opens to allow the chyme to pass into the small intestine. During the next phase of digestion, nutrients from the digested food are absorbed through the intestinal walls and transported throughout the body to provide needed fuel. Waste products (including undigested parts of the food) move into the colon where they remain until feces are expelled by a bowel movement.

What Are Digestive Disorders?

In her book, *Digestive Wellness*, clinical nutritionist Elizabeth Lipski discusses the essential role played by the digestive system in maintaining good health. She writes: “The purpose of the digestive system . . . is to bring nutrients to each cell of your body. When this doesn't occur, we feel tired and sluggish, can't think clearly, and begin to develop symptoms of illness. If left untended, these symptoms can develop into full-blown health problems."[5] The health problems to which Lipski refers are diseases and disorders of the digestive system.

Through years of research, scientists have identified a wide variety of digestive disorders. These range in severity from conditions that are uncomfortable but not particularly serious to those that can be life threatening. One of the most common digestive disorders is heartburn. Washing-

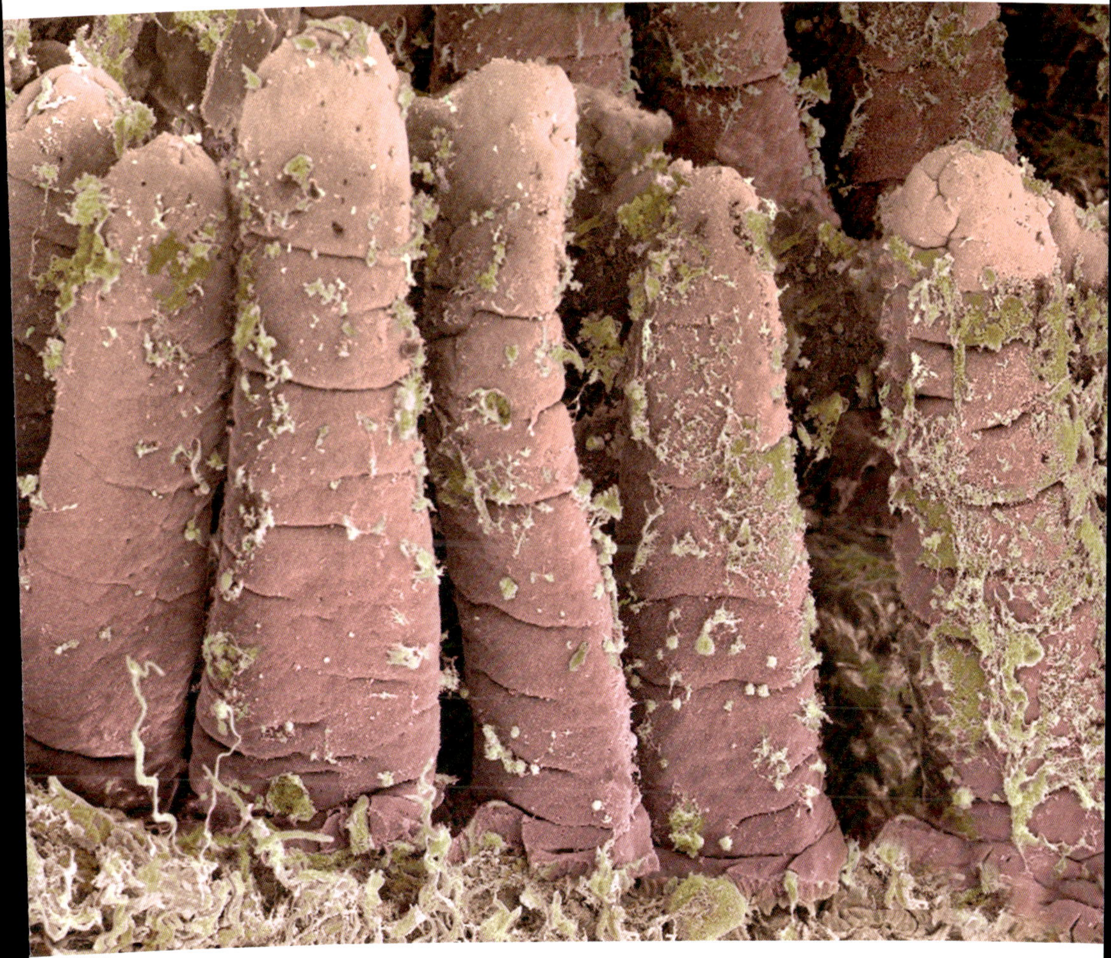

The healthy fingerlike protrusions called villi (pictured in this colored scanning electron micrograph) allow nutrients from food to be absorbed through the walls of the small intestine into the bloodstream. In people with celiac disease, foods containing gluten cause the immune system to damage or destroy the villi.

ton, DC, gastroenterologist Michael Gold describes heartburn as a "hot or burning feeling rising up from the center of the abdomen area and into the chest under the breastbone, or sternum."[6] Chronic heartburn may indicate acid reflux, a condition in which acidic digestive juices flow back up into the esophagus due to the LES's not working properly. The most severe form of acid reflux is known as gastroesophageal reflux disease, or GERD.

> **"Symptoms tend to be especially severe for people with inflammatory bowel disease and often include extremely painful abdominal cramps, poor bowel control, and rectal bleeding."**

Two digestive disorders that involve someone having adverse reactions to certain ingested substances are lactose intolerance and celiac disease. People who suffer from the former have trouble digesting lactose, a natural sugar found in milk and other dairy products. Far more serious is celiac disease, which involves severe intolerance to a protein called gluten that is found in grains such as wheat, barley, and rye. The National Institute of Diabetes and Digestive and Kidney Diseases (NIDDK) writes: "When people with celiac disease eat foods or use products containing gluten, their immune system responds by damaging or destroying villi—the tiny, fingerlike protrusions lining the small intestine. Villi normally allow nutrients from food to be absorbed through the walls of the small intestine into the bloodstream."[7] Without healthy villi, people are deprived of essential nutrients and become malnourished no matter how much food they eat.

Disorders of the Bowel

A number of digestive disorders affect the bowel, one of which is irritable bowel syndrome (IBS). Formerly called spastic colon, IBS is a disorder that affects the muscle contractions of the digestive system. Johns Hopkins Medicine further explains the nature of the disorder: "Because people with IBS have a colon that appears to be normal—that is, there are no structural or biochemical abnormalities explaining the symptoms—IBS is called a 'functional' disorder: The system just doesn't work right."[8]

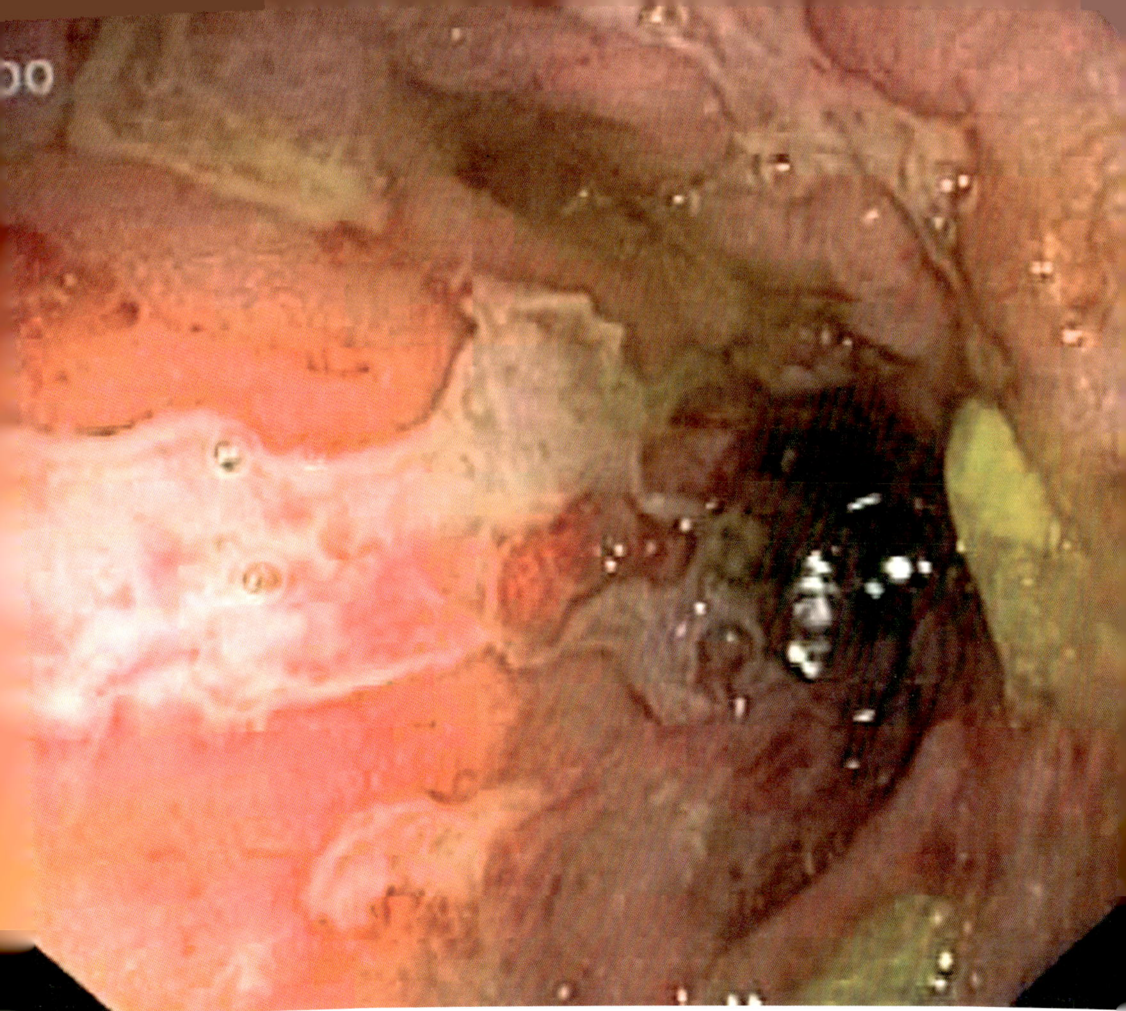

In a patient with Crohn's disease, ulceration and inflammation of the large intestine are visible through an endoscope. Crohn's disease is a digestive disorder characterized by severe abdominal pain and rectal bleeding.

Since the names are similar, IBS is often confused with inflammatory bowel disease, but the disorders are very different. The latter is a broad term referring to chronic inflammation of the gastrointestinal tract and is far more serious and debilitating than IBS. The two main types of inflammatory bowel disease are Crohn's disease and ulcerative colitis. With Crohn's disease, ulcers form deep in the tissue of any part of the digestive tract, which leads to infection and the development of thick scar tissue. Ulcerative colitis also causes ulcers, but they are limited to the large bowel.

Although they have different characteristics, both types of inflammatory bowel disease involve an abnormal response by the body's immune system. The Centers for Disease Control and Prevention (CDC) explains: "Normally, the immune cells protect the body from infection. In people with IBD [inflammatory bowel disease], however, the immune system mistakes food, bacteria, and other materials in the intestine for foreign substances and it attacks the cells of the intestines. In the process, the body sends white blood cells into the lining of the intestines where they produce chronic inflammation."[9]

Warning Signs

Each digestive disorder is unique and has its own set of symptoms. Heartburn could be a symptom of acid reflux or, in more serious cases, a warning sign of GERD. Heartburn may also signify that someone has developed a peptic ulcer, although a more typical symptom is sudden, sharp pains between the breastbone and navel. The Mayo Clinic writes: "Burning pain is the most common peptic ulcer symptom. The pain is caused by the ulcer and is aggravated by stomach acid coming in contact with the ulcerated area."[10] Abdominal pain is also a primary symptom of IBS, as are gassiness and abdominal bloating. Also common in people with IBS are erratic, unpredictable bowel habits: a sufferer may be constipated for days and then be stricken with a severe case of diarrhea.

Symptoms tend to be especially severe for people with inflammatory bowel disease and often include extremely painful abdominal cramps, poor bowel control, and rectal bleeding. A British woman named Jennifer Killick suffers from ulcerative colitis and describes the symptoms as "about as humiliating as they come: crippling pain and diarrhoea full of blood and pus." Killick refers to a particularly bad day when she was traveling in a car with some friends and felt like they would never arrive at their destination. "It took all of my energy and concentration to hold back the floodgates," she says. "As I raced up the stairs to the bathroom, undoing my jeans as I ran and unable even to close the door behind me, I was certain I wouldn't make it. But I did. Most colitis sufferers have stories about times when they weren't so lucky."[11]

Millions of Sufferers

It is difficult for health officials to know exactly how many people are affected by digestive disorders because statistics are compiled using data from reported cases; if people do not seek treatment, they are not in-cluded in prevalence data. The NIDDK estimates that from 60 million to 70 million people in the United States are affected by some type of digestive disorder. Among the most common is heartburn, which affects an estimated 60 million Americans once a month and 15 million on a daily basis. Although people of all ages and walks of life suffer from heartburn, the highest incidence is among pregnant women and the elderly.

> **“Because many digestive disorders have similar symptoms, it is important for patients to seek medical attention rather than trying to diagnose themselves.”**

An estimated 10 million to 15 million Americans suffer from a peptic ulcer. Two to three times that many develop lactose intolerance, with the highest prevalence among blacks, Asians, and Native Americans. According to the Crohn's & Colitis Foundation, more than 1.4 million Americans suffer from inflammatory bowel disease. A study published in 2012 by the Mayo Clinic found that celiac disease affects an estimated 1.8 million Americans, whereas 10 to 15 percent of the US population suffers from irritable bowel syndrome.

Digestive Disorders in Children and Teens

Some types of digestive disorders are as prevalent in children and teenagers as in adults. One example is IBS, which is one of the most common digestive disorders among adolescents. According to the International Foundation for Functional Gastrointestinal Disorders, an estimated 17 percent of high school students and 8 percent of middle school students suffer from IBS. Although inflammatory bowel disease usually strikes young adults in their twenties and thirties, an estimated 20 to 30 percent of sufferers develop it before the age of twenty. According to the Crohn's and Colitis Foundation of America, more than one hundred thousand children and teens in the United States suffer from either Crohn's disease or ulcerative colitis.

One digestive disorder that only affects infants and children is known as Hirschsprung disease, which is characterized by the absence of nerves in parts of the intestine. It affects roughly one in five thousand infants and is a congenital disorder, meaning one that develops before a baby is born. About half of the children with Hirschsprung disease are diagnosed soon after birth, and the rest are usually diagnosed by the time they are two years old.

What Causes Digestive Disorders?

Depending on the type, a number of causes may be involved in the development of digestive disorders, but in many cases scientists cannot pinpoint an exact cause. One example is lactose intolerance; people who suffer from it lack the enzyme lactase, but the reasons for this deficiency are unknown. Another digestive disorder whose cause is puzzling to scientists is GERD. Although it is well known that the LES malfunctions in people with the disorder, no one knows exactly what causes the muscle to become faulty. A known contributing factor, however, is smoking, as people who smoke regularly have a higher incidence of acid reflux than nonsmokers.

Genetics is believed to play a role in a number of digestive disorders. Scientists believe, for instance, that genetic abnormalities (mutations) are at least partly responsible for the development of inflammatory bowel disease. One digestive disorder that is known to have genetic roots is Hirschsprung disease, although that does not necessarily mean that it is hereditary. According to the National Institutes of Health, only about 20 percent of Hirschsprung cases occur in multiple members of the same family, and the remaining cases occur in babies with no family history of the disorder.

Arriving at a Diagnosis

Because many digestive disorders have similar symptoms, it is important for patients to seek medical advice rather than trying to diagnose themselves. Using the example of lactose intolerance, Children's Hospital Boston's Center for Young Women's Health writes: "The same discomfort caused by lactose intolerance can be caused by other conditions, including Crohn's disease, irritable bowel syndrome, and an infection of the small intestine. These conditions can be serious if they are not properly treated. Your health care provider is the only person who can confirm that you are lactose intolerant or if you have another condition."[12]

Diagnosis of any digestive disorder begins with a complete physical examination and medical history. Then, depending on the patient's symptoms, a wide array of tests can help the physician confirm a diagnosis. For example, blood tests can help diagnose celiac disease by detecting high levels of antibodies to gluten. X-rays of the digestive system, which are known as upper or lower GI series, can help diagnose many different disorders. A diagnostic technique known as an endoscopy is a way for a doctor to visually examine the esophagus. He or she uses a thin, flexible instrument known as an endoscope that is fitted with a tiny camera at the end. After the device is threaded through the mouth and down the esophagus, it begins to transmit pictures that the doctor can closely examine for inflammation or bleeding.

What Are the Effects of Digestive Disorders?

Life can be difficult for people with digestive disorders. Just how difficult depends on the severity of the disorder, as the University of Pittsburgh Medical Center (UPMC) Digestive Disorders Center explains: "For some people, digestive disorders cause discomfort, embarrassment, and a loss of work time. For others, these disorders can be extremely serious, ruining their quality of life. They can even be life-threatening."[13]

Although people of all ages suffer from the effects of digestive disorders, teenagers with these disorders can have an especially tough time. They are already coping with the typical challenges associated with adolescence, and having to deal with a chronic illness can seem overwhelming. One teenage girl who knows this from personal experience is Nicolle, who wrote in an online forum in May 2012 about the difficulties of coping with irritable bowel syndrome. "Every day is a constant struggle with IBS," she says. Formally an A student, Nicolle often makes excuses not to go to school out of fear that she will have an attack of severe abdominal cramps followed by diarrhea. When she is at school, she rarely eats anything in an effort to avoid a flare-up. "In other words," she writes,

> **"Although people of all ages suffer from the effects of digestive disorders, teenagers with these disorders can have an especially tough time."**

"I'm afraid that if I eat, my IBS will act up and I'll be stranded in an awfully uncomfortable situation. . . . I just wish this would go away and no one would have to suffer from it."[14]

Prevention Strategies

Not all digestive disorders can be prevented, but experts say that many can be managed and sometimes avoided by adopting healthier lifestyle habits. Referring to chronic heartburn and acid reflux, Mayo Clinic physician Michael F. Picco writes: "Lose excess weight, eat smaller meals, and avoid foods that seem to trigger heartburn—such as fried or fatty foods, chocolate and peppermint. Avoiding alcohol and nicotine may help, too."[15] Exercise, which has innumerable health benefits, can also help prevent many digestive disorders. The combination of regular exercise and a nutritious diet, for instance, can help prevent obesity, which has been connected to a number of digestive problems, including acid reflux. Adopting a healthier lifestyle can also help keep IBS symptoms under control and possibly even eliminate them altogether.

> **"Not all digestive disorders can be prevented, but experts say that many can be managed and sometimes avoided by adopting healthier lifestyle habits."**

Celiac disease is not preventable, but a strict diet that avoids any foods containing gluten can prevent flare-ups. The same is true for lactose intolerance; sufferers can avoid flare-ups by staying away from dairy products and other foods that contain lactose.

How Are Digestive Disorders Treated?

Many digestive disorders are treatable if people seek medical attention. Acid reflux, for example, can often be successfully treated with drugs that reduce acid levels, known as proton pump inhibitors. People with severe cases of GERD may need to undergo fundoplication surgery, which strengthens the natural barrier between the stomach and esophagus. During the operation the surgeon gathers the part of the stomach closest to the entry of the esophagus, wraps it around the lower esophagus, and then sutures it to keep it in place. This increases pressure at the lower end of the esophagus, and thereby prevents digestive acids from refluxing back into it.

Many treatments are also available for IBS. According to the NIDDK, the disorder can often be successfully treated with a combination of diet and medications. Another treatment is probiotics, which are live microbes contained in many different types of products, including foods (such as yogurt), medications, and dietary supplements. These microbes, when ingested, help restore a balanced, healthy condition. In addition, many IBS patients may benefit from psychotherapy because of emotional problems caused by struggling with a chronic illness.

Far Beyond Bellyaches

Millions of people suffer from digestive disorders, which range from occasional heartburn to chronic conditions like inflammatory bowel disease. These disorders can cause many problems for sufferers, both physically and emotionally, and interfere with their quality of life. When diagnosed and treated, however, many people are able to overcome digestive disorders and live normal, healthy lives.

What Are Digestive Disorders?

"There is currently an epidemic of digestive illness in our country, one that is directly related to the foods we eat and the way we live."

Elizabeth Lipski, a clinical nutritionist who is director of doctoral studies at Hawthorn University and author of the book *Digestive Wellness*.

"Every section of the GI tract is prone to its own unique disorder—some are merely annoying, such as heartburn, while others can be painful or even debilitating with cramping, bloating, diarrhea, constipation, or bleeding."

Todd Brown, a doctor of chiropractic medicine from Cumming, Georgia.

After suffering from stomach problems for as long as she could remember, a young woman named Alysa Bajenaru was desperate to find out what was wrong. During the summer of 2011, two years after the birth of her daughter, Bajenaru's pain grew worse, and new symptoms began to appear, as she wrote in her blog: "Much more pain, stomach upset all the time, skin breaking out, brittle nails. My clothes don't fit. I haven't gained any weight, but I am so bloated that sometimes I look 6 months pregnant."[16] Bajenaru had no idea why she was having these symptoms. A professional dietician, she was committed to living a healthy lifestyle by eating right and exercising on a regular basis, but these efforts were no longer working. Something was obviously very wrong.

Bajenaru saw a gastroenterologist and underwent a number of tests, and finally she had an answer: celiac disease. Although she was aware that sticking to a diet completely free of gluten would be challenging, any trace of negativity was overshadowed by the relief of no longer having to wonder what was wrong with her. This optimism was reflected in her blog post of August 11, 2011: "Let me just say that there is no reason to feel bad. This is a time to celebrate! I have already gone almost a week eating gluten-free and this is the best I have felt in a very long time. I am so thankful to have a diagnosis, especially one that is curable with food."[17]

Harsh Reality

Only a few months had passed before Bajenaru's euphoria began to wane, as she found out how challenging it was to cope with celiac disease—so challenging that she wondered why she had ever viewed it as something to feel positive about. She wrote: "The truth is, celiac disease is hard. It is SO hard. I'm a freaking dietician and I can't even handle it."[18] What Bajenaru learned over time is that living with celiac disease involves a great deal more than just watching her diet. She has to be constantly vigilant about every morsel of food she puts in her mouth, and even that is not always enough.

> **Although awareness of celiac disease has soared in recent years, it actually traces back to ancient times.**

In October 2012, for instance, Bajenaru was having dinner at a restaurant and "got glutened," which is how she refers to gluten finding its way into her system. Telltale symptoms started showing up immediately, as she writes: "Tingling brain, pinching sensation in my brain, chills, trouble focusing my eyes, trouble focusing my thoughts, trouble getting complete sentences out." Some of her symptoms lingered for two weeks, including headaches, swelling in her fingers, "short temper, burning scalp, hot flashes, upset stomach, fatigue."[19] A short time afterward Bajenaru accidentally "glutened" herself. She bought popcorn that was labeled as having no gluten but neglected to scrutinize the label on the back. It stated that the popcorn was processed in a facility that also produced wheat products, meaning that the popcorn was cross-contaminated with gluten. After just one handful, Bajenaru suffered the usual severe physical reaction, as she writes: "I sat on the bed with tears streaming down my face. Why did I think it was going to be easy, this celiac living? How could I have celebrated my diagnosis?"[20]

Centuries of Mystery

Although awareness of celiac disease has soared in recent years, it actually traces back to ancient times. As early as the second century AD, scientists were offering their theories about a mysterious digestive condition that made sufferers extremely sick. The ancient Greek physician Aretaeus of Cappadocia, for example, observed that celiac disease led to symptoms such as flatulence (gas) and diarrhea and concluded that it resulted from incomplete digestion of food. In describing one suffering patient, Aretaeus wrote: "Emaciated and atrophied [shrunken], pale, feeble and incapable of performing any of his accustomed works, but if he attempts to walk, the limbs fail, the veins in the temples are prominent, for owing to wasting the temples are hollow, but also all over the body the veins are enlarged."[21]

> **"When people who are lactose intolerant consume milk, cheese, ice cream, or other dairy products that contain lactose, they suffer from symptoms such as flatulence, abdominal cramps, the feeling of being bloated, and diarrhea."**

Hundreds of years later, scientists were still proposing theories about celiac disease. Many correctly deduced that it was related to diet, but no one could identify the culprit. In 1924 an American pediatrician named Sidney Valentine Haas described how he had successfully treated eight children whom he had diagnosed with celiac disease. He fed them a banana diet and intentionally excluded bread, crackers, potatoes, and cereals. Although Haas was convinced that the healing resulted from the bananas, experts later concluded that his success with the patients actually came from the elimination of gluten-containing grains.

One of the first to propose gluten as the root of celiac disease was Dutch pediatrician Willem-Karel Dicke. He had become curious in the early 1930s about the link between wheat and celiac disease after consulting with a mother whose young child suffered from a severe skin rash. The mother explained to Dicke that when she removed bread and biscuits from the child's diet, the child improved rapidly. Intrigued by this, Dicke went on to conduct experiments with celiac disease patients by feeding them wheat-free diets, and he was encouraged by the results. He wrote about these and other observations in a 1950 thesis titled *Investigation of the Harmful Effects of Certain Types of Cereal on Patients with Coeliac Disease.*

No Tolerance for Dairy

Millions of people throughout the world suffer from lactose intolerance, a disorder that results from a deficiency of an enzyme called lactase. Produced in the digestive tract, lactase's function is to convert the lactose, or milk sugar, in dairy products into simple sugars that the body can use for energy. When people who are lactose intolerant consume milk, cheese, ice cream, or other dairy products, they suffer from symptoms such as flatulence, abdominal cramps, the feeling of being bloated, and diarrhea. The German Institute for Quality and Efficiency in Health Care explains: "These symptoms are usually linked to the amount of lactose the person has consumed: small amounts do not usually cause symptoms at all, while very large amounts can cause symptoms."[22]

> **"Research has consistently shown that gastroesophageal reflux (GER) is among the most common digestive disorders."**

A twenty-one-year-old woman named Sandra suffers from lactose intolerance and says she has a difficult struggle with it. She is Italian, loves Italian food, and her favorite dishes all contain cheese—which because of her disorder, she cannot have. Eating in restaurants is often tricky because it is difficult for Sandra to find meals that are completely free of dairy products. "For example," she says, "there's a restaurant chain in Canada called Moxies and their tomato sauce has [parmesan] cheese in it. Who would have thought?"[23]

Sandra says that having to live with a diet that is radically different from what she has long been used to is tough. "Sometimes I get distraught," she says. "I always ate dairy and to suddenly alter your diet is very hard." For the most part, though, she manages to keep a positive attitude and has words of hope for others who suffer from lactose intolerance: "There are lots of books, resources to help you out. Friends, family are there. The one thing I have picked up is that I now cook really well because I am constantly trying to create dairy-free recipes."[24]

A Product of the Mind?

According to Mary Maish, who is surgical director of the Center for Esophageal Disorders at the University of California–Los Angeles, many people who think they are lactose intolerant actually suffer from unaddressed psychological issues. But that does not necessarily mean that they are imagining their problems, as Maish explains: "It's a real thing, they really do have these symptoms."[25] In May 2011, a study announced by a team of researchers from the University of Milan in Italy reinforced Maish's perspective about psychological rather than physical reasons for the disorder.

The study, led by gastroenterologist Guido Basilisco, involved more than a hundred people. All had been suffering from symptoms such as stomach pain, bloating, and diarrhea, and all believed that they were lactose intolerant. Participants underwent breath tests that are commonly used to diagnose lactose intolerance. They were also questioned about their mental and physical health, including whether they suffered from depression, anxiety, and/or general aches and pains. At the conclusion of the study, the team found that less than one-third of the participants actually suffered from lactose intolerance. The physical symptoms experienced by the remainder of patients were likely due to a somatoform disorder, in which a person's symptoms are caused by psychological problems rather than by a physical condition.

According to Basilisco, the study's findings illustrate why people should not necessarily assume they suffer from lactose intolerance when they experience similar symptoms. He stresses that physicians need to be aware of this and urge patients not to be so quick to eliminate dairy products—which contain essential nutrients such as calcium—from their diets. "Excluding dairy products should be discouraged," says Basilisco, "and doctors should pay more attention to the psychological problems of their patients."[26]

Acid Reflux

Research has consistently shown that gastroesophageal reflux (GER) is among the most common digestive disorders. The condition is most often referred to as acid reflux because digestive acid backs up along with food into the esophagus when the LES is not working properly. The word *reflux* comes from the medieval Latin word *refluxus*, which is derived from the Latin word *refluere*, meaning "to flow back or recede." The NIDDK describes the condition:

"When acid reflux occurs, food or fluid can be tasted in the back of the mouth. When refluxed stomach acid touches the lining of the esophagus it may cause a burning sensation in the chest or throat called heartburn or acid indigestion. Occasional GER is common and does not necessarily mean one has GERD. Persistent reflux that occurs more than twice a week is considered GERD."[27]

> **Throughout the world millions of people of all ages and all walks of life are affected by digestive disorders.**

In December 2011, a team of researchers from Norway released a long-term study that involved tracking the digestive health of nearly thirty thousand people. The team found that the prevalence of acid reflux rose 30 percent over the study period, with incidence of severe acid reflux rising 24 percent. One of the most profound findings was that the number of people who were troubled by acid reflux at least once per week increased nearly 50 percent between 1995 and 2009. In the follow-up report, the study authors write: "The present study found a substantial increase in the prevalence of GORS [gastro-oesophageal reflux symptoms] during the past decade."[28]

One Teen's Battle

A teenager from New York City named Isaac J. Kassin has struggled with GERD for several years. The first symptom he noticed was discomfort in his chest after eating, as he explains: "I felt an acidic burn that pierced . . . my chest, and then sharply burned my esophagus, a pain lasting for 24 hours seven days a week. After a while my entire chest and stomach went tight, and my breathing was stifled. My esophagus was also sore, and the constant burning irritated it."[29] Kassin underwent a series of tests and learned that the GERD had resulted from celiac disease, which he never knew he had.

Immediately, Kassin's doctor put him on a strict diet, as he explains: "I wasn't allowed to eat anything with gluten, wheat, dairy, or acid, even on a microscopic level. My body simply couldn't digest them. When I did, I suffered the consequences: painful periods of acid reflux, long indigestion, and a full day of heartburn."[30] Kassin found the restricted eating to be challenging as well as frustrating, largely because he was hungry all the time and felt like he was "starving to death." He writes: "It was a hard transition to not only stop eating all foods that contained the products I couldn't eat, but also avoid the products that I feared would bring on the pain. It was extra hard when I went out with my friends. This led and sometimes still does lead to sleepless nights due to sadness."[31]

No Fun Whatsoever

Throughout the world millions of people of all ages and all walks of life are affected by digestive disorders. These conditions range from celiac disease, in which sufferers cannot tolerate even a trace of gluten, to lactose intolerance, heartburn, and such painful acid reflux that people feel like their chests are on fire. Much about these illnesses remains unknown, but through ongoing research scientists continue to learn more about them. This growing body of knowledge will keep expanding throughout the coming years, which means there may be more hope than ever for digestive disorder sufferers.

Primary Source Quotes*

What Are Digestive Disorders?

“‘Heartburn’ has nothing to do with the heart, but is the burning sensation produced by acid reflux into the esophagus.”

Kenneth S. Saladin, *Anatomy & Physiology*. New York: McGraw-Hill Education, 2010, p. 975.

Saladin is a distinguished professor of biology at Georgia College and State University.

“Ulcers often come and go spontaneously without the individual ever knowing that they are present unless a serious complication (like bleeding or perforation) occurs.”

Jay W. Marks, “Peptic Ulcer Disease,” MedicineNet, May 16, 2012. www.medicinenet.com.

Marks is an internist and gastroenterologist in Mission Viejo, California.

---

* Editor's Note: While the definition of a primary source can be narrowly or broadly defined, for the purposes of Compact Research, a primary source consists of: 1) results of original research presented by an organization or researcher; 2) eyewitness accounts of events, personal experience, or work experience; 3) first-person editorials offering pundits' opinions; 4) government officials presenting political plans and/or policies; 5) representatives of organizations presenting testimony or policy.

“When people with celiac disease eat foods containing gluten, their immune systems respond by attacking and damaging the lining of the small intestine. The small intestine is responsible for absorbing nutrients from food into the bloodstream for the body to use.”

National Institutes of Health (NIH), “What People with Celiac Disease Need to Know About Osteoporosis,” January 2012. www.niams.nih.gov.

The NIH is an agency of the US Department of Health and Human Services and the largest source of medical research funding in the world.

“Ulcerative colitis is a chronic disease of the digestive tract where symptoms tend to come and go.”

University of Maryland Medical Center, “Turmeric,” May 4, 2011.

The University of Maryland Medical Center is a teaching hospital in Baltimore, Maryland.

“The occurrence of irritable bowel syndrome (IBS) in children is similar to the rate in adults.”

International Foundation for Functional Gastrointestinal Disorders (IFFGD), “Kids & Teens,” August 22, 2012. www.iffgd.org.

The IFFGD is an education and research organization that seeks to inform, assist, and support people who are affected by gastrointestinal disorders.

“In Crohn’s disease, all layers of the intestine may be involved and there can be normal healthy bowel between patches of diseased bowel.”

Centers for Disease Control and Prevention (CDC), “Inflammatory Bowel Disease,” May 1, 2012. www.cdc.gov.

The CDC is a federal agency dedicated to protecting health and promoting quality of life through the prevention and control of disease, injury, and disability.

"People with a functional GI disorder have frequent symptoms, but the GI tract does not become damaged."

National Institute of Diabetes and Digestive and Kidney Diseases (NIDDK), "Irritable Bowel Syndrome," July 2, 2012. http://digestive.niddk.nih.gov.

The NIDDK conducts and supports medical research and research training to improve the health and quality of life of people suffering from diabetes and digestive and kidney diseases.

"People who are lactose intolerant have problems such as nausea, stomach cramps, gas, bloating, and diarrhea after they eat or drink milk or foods that contain lactose."

Center for Young Women's Health at Boston Children's Hospital, "Lactose Intolerance," September 29, 2011. www.youngwomenshealth.org.

The Center for Young Women's Health at Boston Children's Hospital is one of the largest pediatric medical centers in the United States.

"Symptoms of heartburn, also known as acid indigestion, are more common among the elderly and pregnant women."

American College of Gastroenterology, "Acid Reflux," 2012. http://patients.gi.org.

Composed of more than twelve thousand physicians, the American College of Gastroenterology seeks to advance the medical treatment and scientific study of gastrointestinal disorders.

What Are Digestive Disorders?

- The National Institute of Diabetes and Digestive and Kidney Diseases (NIDDK) states that **60 million to 70 million** people in the United States are affected by digestive disorders.
- According to the Centers for Disease Control and Prevention (CDC), up to **1.4 million** Americans suffer from inflammatory bowel disease.
- A report released in August 2012 by the Mayo Clinic states that celiac disease affects **1.8 million** Americans.
- According to the American College of Gastroenterology, more than **15 million** Americans experience heartburn on a daily basis.
- According to Harvard Medical School, irritable bowel syndrome affects approximately **24 million** people in the United States, **70 percent** of whom are women.
- A 2010 report by researchers from Sweden states that up to **25 percent** of patients with inflammatory bowel disease developed it during childhood or adolescence.
- According to University of Wisconsin School of Medicine physician Arnold Wald, at least **2.5 million** doctor visits in the United States each year are due to constipation, and hundreds of millions of dollars are spent on laxatives.

Facts and Illustrations

Prevalence Varies Widely

Researchers have identified numerous diseases and disorders that affect the digestive system. Chronic constipation and gastroesophageal reflux disease (GERD) are the most prevalent, whereas inflammatory bowel diseases are far less common.

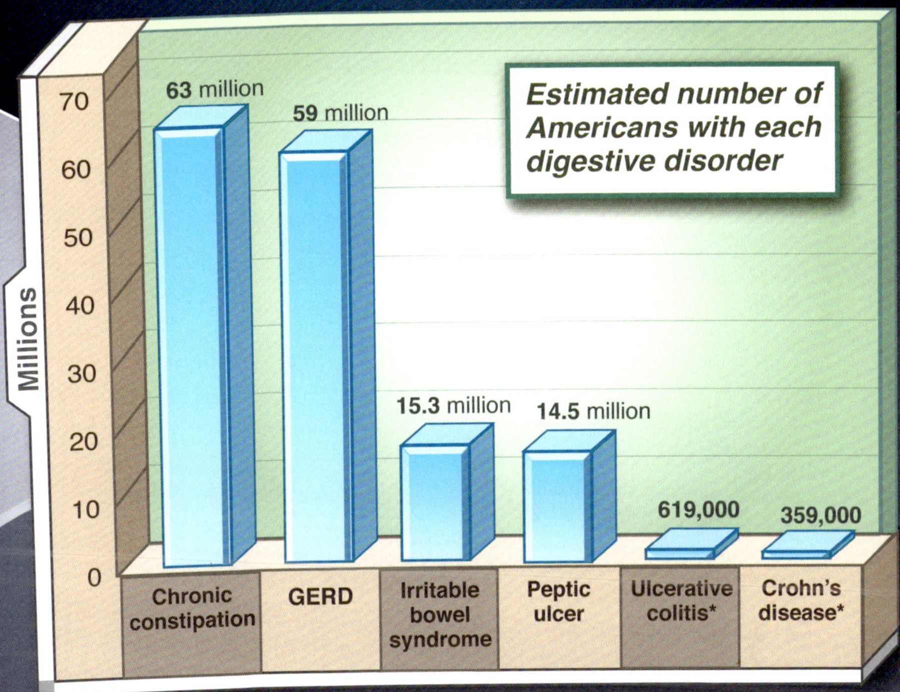

*Ulcerative colitis and Crohn's disease are the two major types of inflammatory bowel disease.

Source: National Institute of Diabetes and Digestive and Kidney Diseases, "Digestive Disease Statistics for the United States," May 10, 2012. http://digestive.niddk.nih.gov.

- Registered dietician Maria A. Bella says that two out of three adults aged sixty-five and older experience **acid reflux.**
- The CDC estimates that **10 percent** of inflammatory bowel disease cases occur in adolescents under eighteen years of age.

Dairy, Gluten Most Common Food Intolerances

During a survey conducted in May 2012, more than nine hundred subscribers to a website that educates people about food intolerance were asked about their personal experience with it. Nearly 70 percent said they suffered from one or more types. The most common food intolerances were dairy products and the protein known as gluten.

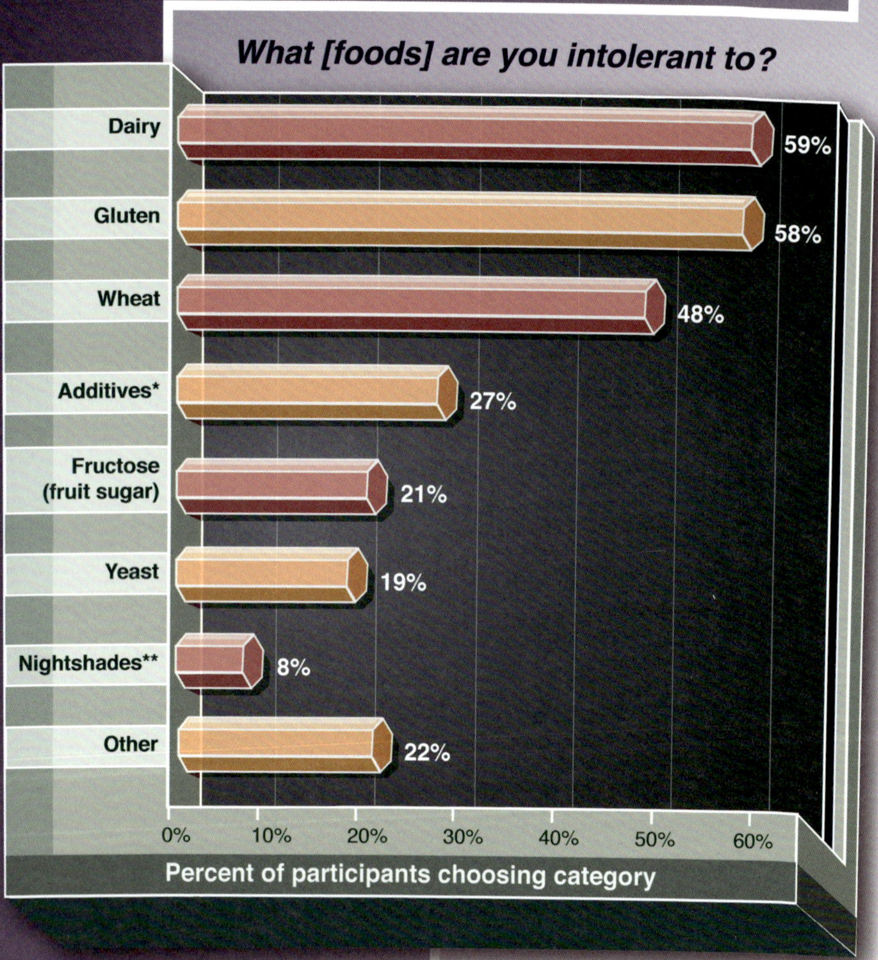

* Additives are substances added to food to preserve or enhance flavor and appearance.

** Nightshades comprise a diverse family of plants that include potatoes, tomatoes, sweet and hot peppers, and eggplant.

Note: Participants could choose more than one category, so total exceeds 100 percent.

Source: Food Intolerance Institute of Australia, "The Foodintol Survey 2012," December 4, 2012. www.foodintol.com.

Acid Reflux Prevalence Growing

Acid reflux is defined as the backwash of digestive acids into the esophagus from the stomach, a disorder that affects tens of millions of people. When researchers from Norway analyzed the prevalence of acid reflux among a large group of adults between 1995 and 1997, and between 2006 and 2009 they found that prevalence has increased over the years. They did not identify a specific reason for the increase.

Prevalence of acid reflux symptoms: 1995–1997 and 2006–2009

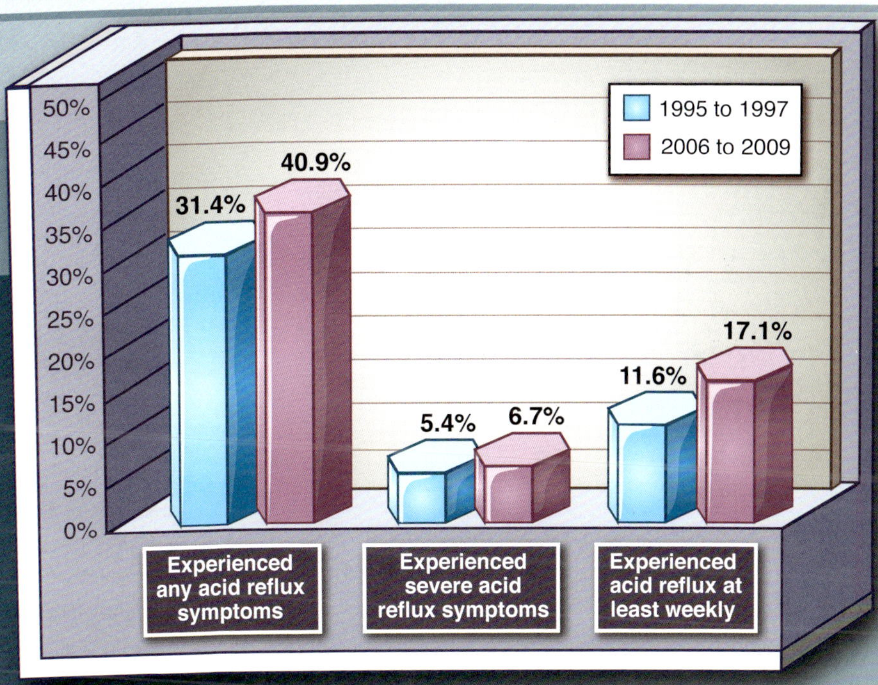

Source: Eivind Ness-Jensen et al, "Changes in Prevalence, Incidence and Spontaneous Loss of Gastro-Oesophageal Reflux Symptoms: A Prospective Population-Based Cohort Study, the HUNT Study," *Gut*, December 22, 2011. www.ntnu.edu.

- According to pediatrician Andrew B. Grossman, an estimated **one hundred thousand** teens and preteens have Crohn's disease.

- The NIDDK states that about a **half-million** people in the United States develop a peptic ulcer each year.

What Causes Digestive Disorders?

"Both genetics and early life experiences influence an individual's susceptibility to adult functional gastrointestinal disorders."

International Foundation for Functional Gastrointestinal Disorders, an educational and research organization that seeks to inform, assist, and support people who are affected by digestive disorders.

"Nutrition is inseparably intertwined with disorders of digestion."

Bhaskar Banerjee, chief of gastroenterology and professor of medicine at the University of Arizona College of Medicine.

Until the latter part of the twentieth century, the prevailing scientific belief about ulcers was that they were caused by turmoil in people's lives—namely, too much stress. This was based on the theory that when people were stressed out their digestive systems produced excess stomach acid, which led to the development of gastritis (inflammation of the stomach) and then an ulcer. The theory was incorrect but rarely challenged, as Australian scientist Barry J. Marshall explains: "There was this idea that stress caused high acid levels; maybe there was a small amount of evidence for that, although I haven't been able to find it when I've looked. Anyway, all those things added up to convince people that ulcers were caused by stress. . . . It was smoke and mirrors as much as anything else, but terribly convincing for everybody."[32]

In the 1880s some German researchers proposed that the real cause of ulcers might be bacteria, but that notion was flatly rejected by their peers. Scientists worldwide were convinced that the stomach was far too acidic an environment for any type of bacteria to survive. Even a hundred years later those beliefs remained unchanged and were rarely challenged. So in 1981, when Marshall and his colleague J. Robin Warren reintroduced the possibility that bacteria caused ulcers, it was not surprising when they encountered major skepticism—and ridicule—from their fellow scientists.

Refuting Conventional Beliefs

After years of research, Warren and Marshall had arrived at the conclusion that ulcers developed not as a result of stress, but because of infection with a type of bacteria called *Helicobacter pylori* (*H. pylori*). In a June 1984 article in the British medical journal *The Lancet* they described one of their studies, in which they found a clear connection between the corkscrew-shaped *H. pylori* and ulcers. Of the patients who participated, all those with duodenal ulcers (ulcers of the duodenum, or first 12 inches [30.5 cm] of the small intestine) and nearly all with gastric (stomach) ulcers were found to be infected with the bacteria.

> **"In 1981, when two Australian physicians reintroduced the possibility that bacteria caused ulcers, it was not surprising when they encountered major skepticism—and ridicule—from their fellow scientists."**

After the article was published, most scientists still remained unconvinced and continued to denounce the idea that ulcers were caused by bacteria. This was extremely frustrating for Warren and Marshall. They knew that as long as people clung to incorrect theories, patients would not be successfully treated for ulcers. So Marshall decided that a radical move was in order, as he explains: "The skeptics were so determinedly skeptical that I felt like: I'm never going to prove to these guys that the bacteria are harmful. . . . So I took some bacteria off a patient and cooked it up."[33] By "cooked it up," Marshall is referring to a bold—and dangerous—action on his part. As the ultimate test of *H. pylori*'s role in the development of ulcers, he gathered a large quantity of the bacteria and swallowed it.

For five days Marshall remained symptom free, and then he was stricken with severe nausea and vomiting. An endoscopy revealed that he had developed gastritis, and further tests confirmed that he was positive for *H. pylori* infection. When treatment with antibiotics cleared up his inflammation, there was no longer any doubt that bacteria could indeed survive in the stomach and cause ulcers. Amazingly, however, even that was not enough, and many scientists continued to be skeptical and remained so for more than a decade.

> **"Studies have shown that people with a family history of inflammatory bowel disease have a higher risk of developing it themselves, which strongly suggests genetic ties."**

Through years of extensive research, a great deal has been learned about *H. pylori* and its role in ulcer formation. One issue that remains puzzling to scientists, though, is why about 75 percent of people who are infected with the bacteria never develop ulcers. The NIDDK writes: "Why the bacterium causes ulcers in some people and not in others is not known. Most likely, development of ulcers depends on characteristics of the infected person; the type, or strain, of *H. pylori* present; and factors researchers have yet to discover."[34]

The Role of Stress

Although scientists today widely accept that stress does not cause ulcers, people whose lives are extremely stressful are at risk for a number of digestive problems. Says gastroenterologist Kenneth Koch: "Stress can affect every part of the digestive system." He goes on to say that severe stress can lead to spasms in the esophagus, as well as inflammation in the digestive tract and indigestion. "Under stress," says Koch, "the mill in your stomach can shut down and make you feel nauseous. Stress can cause your colon to react in a way that gives you diarrhea or constipation. We are all familiar with the athlete or the student who has to rush to the bathroom before the big game or the big exam." Koch adds that although stress does not *cause* disorders such as ulcers, celiac disease, or inflammatory bowel disease, "it can make these and other diseases of digestion worse."[35]

One digestive disorder that has been closely linked to stress is irritable bowel syndrome. According to the NIDDK, stress can stimulate colon spasms in people who suffer from IBS: "The colon has many nerves that connect it to the brain. These nerves control the normal contractions of the colon and cause abdominal discomfort at stressful times. In people with IBS, the colon can be overly responsive to even slight conflict or stress. Stress makes the mind more aware of the sensations that arise in the colon."[36] The NIDDK goes on to say that this can become a vicious cycle: IBS symptoms make a person feel more stressed, which in turn intensifies symptoms.

Genetics + Environment

On a web page titled "What Causes Inflammatory Bowel Diseases (IBD)?," the University of North Carolina at Chapel Hill School of Medicine mentions one of the few certainties about inflammatory bowel disease: that despite prolific research, the cause remains unknown. The authors go on to explain that "these chronically recurring episodes of inflammation in the human bowel are related to a complex interaction between various environmental factors and a hereditary predisposition for these diseases."[37]

> **"As with most digestive disorders, scientists have no simple answers to the question of what causes irritable bowel syndrome."**

With regard to heredity, studies have shown that people with a family history of inflammatory bowel disease have a higher risk of developing it themselves, which strongly suggests genetic ties. Researchers have identified certain genes that are likely involved in the development of Crohn's disease and ulcerative colitis. Heredity is only one piece of a complicated puzzle, however. Since most people with genetic vulnerability do not develop inflammatory bowel disease, environmental factors must also be involved. The University of North Carolina article explains: "It is clear that this hereditary predisposition alone cannot lead to the outbreak of disease: this requires the presence of further, as yet unidentified, factors."[38]

Physicians who specialize in digestive disorders emphasize that smoking is one of the main environmental factors connected with inflammatory bowel disease. The exact reason for this connection is unknown, but as the NIDDK explains: "Some researchers believe that smoking might lower the intestines' defenses, decrease blood flow to the intestines, or cause immune system changes that result in inflammation."[39] Examining the link between smoking and inflammatory bowel disease was the focus of a study published in September 2012. A team of researchers from Boston Children's Hospital and Harvard Medical School collected information from nearly 230,000 female nurses who had been involved in comprehensive health studies. The team found that smokers were 90 percent more likely to develop Crohn's disease than were women who had never smoked.

> **"Scientists are aggressively pursuing research in an effort to find answers to the causes of [celiac] disease because its prevalence has soared over the past sixty years."**

The Downside of Antibiotics

For many years scientists and health officials have cautioned people that antibiotics are not a cure-all and should only be taken when they can be effective. For instance, these medications cannot cure viruses that cause the common cold and flu, yet they are often prescribed anyway. Excessive use of antibiotics is risky because it can destroy beneficial bacteria in the digestive tract, which increases vulnerability to infection and illness. According to a study published in September 2012, the overuse of antibiotics by children is contributing to a rising incidence of pediatric inflammatory bowel disease.

A team of researchers from Seattle, Washington, and Philadelphia, Pennsylvania, followed more than a million children who were enrolled in a United Kingdom health registry. Nearly 750 of the children suffered from some form of inflammatory bowel disease. The team found that those treated with antibiotics before their first birthday were more than five times more likely to develop either Crohn's disease or ulcerative colitis than the children who were never treated with antibiotics. Says Ilseung Cho, a gastroenterology expert from New York University's Langone Medical Center: "Both physicians and parents are at fault for the overuse of antibiotics. Antibiotics are very beneficial drugs, but it is important to be prudent about how we use them."[40]

A Cluster of Causes

As with most digestive disorders, scientists have no simple answer to the question of what causes irritable bowel syndrome. According to the NIDDK, it is widely believed that a combination of physical and mental factors can lead to the development of the disorder. One possible physical contributor is the interruption of signals between the brain and nerves of the small and large intestines, as the NIDDK explains: "Problems with brain-gut signals may cause IBS symptoms, such as changes in bowel habits and pain or discomfort."[41]

Psychological factors have also been implicated in the development of IBS. In November 2011, for instance, Mayo Clinic researchers released a study that found a strong connection between the disorder and personal trauma. The study involved extensive interviews with more than twenty-six hundred adults who were asked about past traumatic events such as the death of a loved one, a car accident, house fire, physical or mental abuse, or surviving a natural disaster. The research team found that participants who reported severe trauma in their lives had a much higher incidence of IBS than those who had not experienced such trauma.

The Many Mysteries of Celiac Disease

Of all the digestive disorders that are known to exist, none is more perplexing than celiac disease. Scientists are aggressively pursuing research in an effort to find answers to the causes of the disease because its prevalence has soared over the past sixty years. Mayo Clinic researchers suspect that the increase is related to agricultural modifications that have been made to wheat in order to boost its protein content. Says Mayo gastroenterologist Joseph A. Murray: "People aren't born with this. Something triggers it, and with this dramatic rise in all ages, it must be something pervasive in the environment."[42]

Murray was the lead researcher for a study that examined the long-term effects of celiac disease, and involved identifying people who lived for decades with undiagnosed gluten intolerance. He was fortunate enough to locate a collection of blood samples that had been taken from US Air Force recruits during the early 1950s amid concern about outbreaks of bacterial infection. The samples had been preserved in ice over the years so they were intact, and they provided Murray's team with a rare opportunity to perform a long-term analysis.

The team tested the decades-old blood samples for gluten antibodies. They assumed that the positive rate for celiac disease would be the same as it is today, about 1 percent. The number of positive results was much smaller, however, which indicated that celiac disease was exceedingly rare during the 1950s. The researchers compared those results with two recently collected sets from a county in Minnesota. One set of samples was taken from men who were the same age as the air force recruits. The researchers found that these elderly men were four times likelier to have celiac disease than their contemporaries who had been tested fifty years before. The second set of samples was taken from young men who were the same age as the recruits had been at the time their blood was drawn in the 1950s. From these samples, the researchers were able to deduce that young people today are more than four times likelier to have celiac disease than the 1950s recruits.

More Questions than Answers

For more than a century researchers have been studying digestive disorders. A great deal has been accomplished in that time, such as the discovery that ulcers are caused by bacteria and the various genetic and environmental factors that play a role in other diseases of the digestive system. With all that scientists have learned, however, many questions remain, and much more work needs to be done in the coming years to answer them.

Primary Source Quotes*

What Causes Digestive Disorders?

"In the last 10 years, there has been an explosion of scientific discoveries related to the genetic and environmental causes of Crohn's disease."

David Rubin and Corey Siegel, "New Treatments Offer Hope for Crohn's Patients," CNN, August 15, 2012. www.cnn.com.

Rubin is codirector of the University of Chicago's Inflammatory Bowel Disease Center, and Siegel is director of the Inflammatory Bowel Disease Center at Dartmouth-Hitchcock Medical Center in New Hampshire.

"Stress can have a major impact on digestive diseases. For example, increased stress can trigger a flare in Crohn's disease, colitis, and irritable bowel syndrome."

Raymond Cross, "Avoiding Digestive Health Problems," University of Maryland Medical Center, February 4, 2010. www.umm.edu.

Cross is director of the University of Maryland Medical Center's Inflammatory Bowel Disease Program and codirector of the Digestive Health Center.

---

* Editor's Note: While the definition of a primary source can be narrowly or broadly defined, for the purposes of Compact Research, a primary source consists of: 1) results of original research presented by an organization or researcher; 2) eyewitness accounts of events, personal experience, or work experience; 3) first-person editorials offering pundits' opinions; 4) government officials presenting political plans and/or policies; 5) representatives of organizations presenting testimony or policy.

"Inflammatory bowel diseases result from an exaggerated immune response to what would be normal bacteria in someone who has different genes."

Elizabeth Lipski, *Digestive Wellness*. New York: McGraw-Hill, 2012, p. 91.

Lipski is a clinical nutritionist and director of doctoral studies at Hawthorn University.

"Although there's no proven link between stress and acid reflux, stress can be related to increased incidence of acid reflux."

Maria A. Bella, *The Complete Idiot's Guide to the Acid Reflux Diet*. New York: Penguin, 2012, p. 15.

Bella is a registered dietician in New York City.

"Pregnancy and many medications can bring on heartburn or make it worse."

University of Maryland Medical Center, "Heartburn—Overview," January 31, 2011. www.umm.edu.

The University of Maryland Medical Center is a teaching hospital in Baltimore, Maryland.

"The exact cause of irritable bowel syndrome is not known. However, tremendous advances in our understanding of this common and disabling disorder have been made in the last 10 years."

American College of Gastroenterology, "Irritable Bowel Syndrome," 2012. http://patients.gi.org.

Composed of more than twelve thousand physicians, the American College of Gastroenterology seeks to advance the medical treatment and scientific study of gastrointestinal disorders.

"Smoking increases someone's risk of getting an ulcer because the nicotine in cigarettes causes the stomach to produce more acid."

American Academy of Family Physicians, "Ulcers," September 2012. http://kidshealth.org.

The American Academy of Family Physicians represents more than one hundred thousand family physicians, medical residents, and medical students.

"It's a myth that spicy foods or a stressful job can cause peptic ulcers."

Mayo Clinic, "Peptic Ulcer," January 6, 2011. www.mayoclinic.com.

The Mayo Clinic is a world-renowned medical facility headquartered in Rochester, Minnesota.

"People with [ulcerative colitis] have abnormalities of the immune system, but whether these problems are a cause or a result of the disease is still unclear."

The National Institute of Diabetes and Digestive and Kidney Diseases (NIDDK), "Ulcerative Colitis," November 15, 2011. http://digestive.niddk.nih.gov.

The NIDDK conducts and supports medical research and research training to improve the health and quality of life of people suffering from diabetes and digestive and kidney diseases.

What Causes Digestive Disorders?

- Florida gastroenterologist Kenneth R. DeVault states that the most consistent reason for the development of gastroesophageal reflux disease (GERD) is being **overweight**.

- According to the National Institute of Diabetes and Digestive and Kidney Diseases, past **physical or sexual abuse** has been shown to be a factor in whether someone develops irritable bowel syndrome.

- Gastroenterologist Jay W. Marks states that **cigarette smoking** not only causes ulcers, it is also a leading cause of the failure of treatment for ulcers.

- According to Mayo Clinic researcher Yuri Saito-Loftus, child abuse has been shown to be a factor in up to **50 percent** of patients with irritable bowel syndrome.

- In June 2012 researchers at Cedars-Sinai Inflammatory Bowel and Immunobiology Research Institute announced that they had found a link between **certain types of fungi** in the large intestine and the development of inflammatory bowel diseases such as ulcerative colitis.

- According to the Boston Children's Hospital, some people develop **lactose intolerance** after having surgery or a gastrointestinal infection.

- A study released in October 2012 by researchers from Australia found that certain types of **bacteria** may cause and maintain Crohn's disease.

Causes of Ulcers

Peptic ulcers, or open sores that form in the digestive tract, develop when digestive acids eat away at the inner surface of the esophagus, stomach, or small intestine. Although the digestive tract is coated with a layer of mucous that protects it against acid, if the amount of acid increases or mucous decreases, an ulcer can develop. The various causes are shown here.

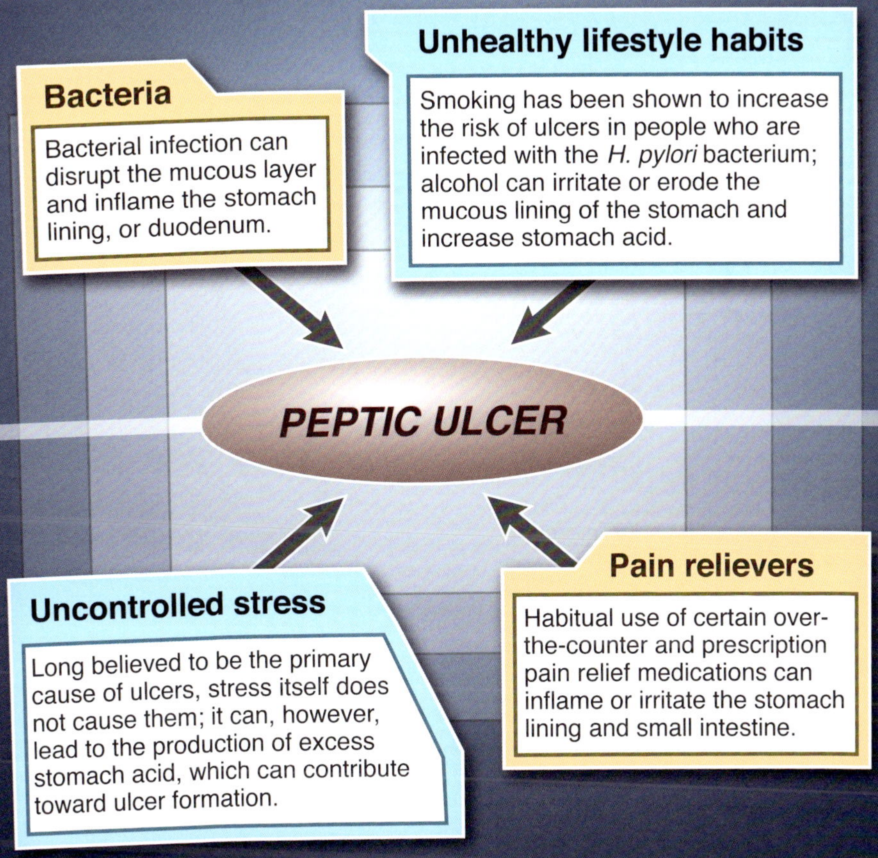

Source: Mayo Clinic, "Peptic Ulcer," January 6, 2011. www.mayoclinic.com.

- According to the Centers for Disease Control and Prevention (CDC), there is strong evidence that **inflammatory bowel disease** is hereditary.

Diet a Strong Factor in GERD

To better understand the effects of gastroesophageal reflux disease (GERD) and associated heartburn on people's lives, the American Gastroenterological Association sponsored a nationwide survey. According to findings released in March 2011, most sufferers report that their symptoms are triggered by dietary habits, especially certain types of food.

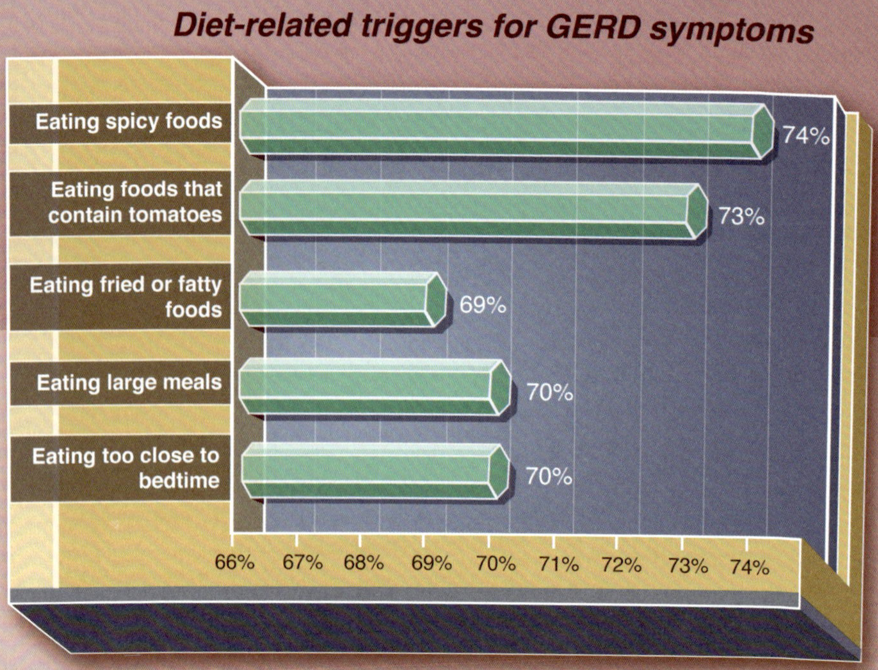

Source: American Gastroenterological Association, "New Nationwide Survey Identifies Need for Increased Dialogue Between Gastroesophageal Reflux Disease or Frequent Heartburn Sufferers and Health Care Providers," March 23, 2011. www.gastro.org.

- According to Johns Hopkins Medicine, *Helicobacter pylori* bacteria cause **90 percent** of all duodenal ulcers and **80 percent** of all gastric ulcers.

- Pediatrician Andrew B. Grossman states that mutations in a gene called CARD15 are present in about **40 percent** of people with Crohn's disease.

The Many Causes of Chronic Constipation

Constipation, which is defined as difficulty emptying the bowels, is one of the most common gastrointestinal complaints. According to the National Institute of Diabetes and Digestive and Kidney Diseases, more than 4 million Americans suffer from frequent constipation, accounting for 2.5 million physician visits each year. Causes vary widely, as shown on this diagram.

Not enough fiber (such as fruits, vegetables, and grains) in the diet
Lack of physical activity (especially in the elderly)
Medications (such as pain relievers, antacids, blood pressure drugs, and others)
Milk
Irritable bowel syndrome
Changes (such as pregnancy, aging, travel) in life or routine
Overuse/abuse of laxatives
Ignoring the urge to have a bowel movement (especially common in young children)
Dehydration
Specific diseases or conditions
Problems with the colon and rectum
Problems with intestinal function

What Are the Effects of Digestive Disorders?

"For some people, digestive disorders cause discomfort, embarrassment, and a loss of work time. For others, these disorders can be extremely serious, ruining their quality of life."

UMPC Digestive Disorders Center, a University of Pittsburgh medical facility that specializes in diseases and disorders that affect the digestive system.

"Though we all suffer differently with celiac disease, we all suffer."

Alysa Bajenaru, a registered dietician who was diagnosed with celiac disease in 2011.

For twenty years, Sophie Lee has fought an agonizing battle with irritable bowel syndrome. Her nightmare began when she was twelve years old and developed a case of food poisoning so severe that she "never really recovered," adding that "whatever happened to my bowel that day transformed a perfectly normal digestive system into an instrument of torture." Over the years Lee has been plagued by numerous symptoms including diarrhea, constipation, bloating, intense abdominal pain, and spasms. One of the worst problems was the unpredictability of her bowels, as she explains: "I would go for days without a bowel movement and then be stuck in the bathroom for an hour."[43]

Eventually Lee discovered a new diet and treatment regimen that worked for her. Yet even with improvements in her physical health, she still continued to struggle with emotional pain, largely because of the dismissive attitudes she encountered from others who were not understanding about her illness. "People thought that IBS was a minor inconvenience, or 'all in your head,' or cured by cutting out coffee," she says. "They thought that it was disgusting and not to be mentioned. They thought that it was shameful." As a way of working through her emotional turmoil, Lee decided to "come out of the IBS closet" and write a book about her experience. "The embarrassed silence that has surrounded IBS for so long needs to be broken," she says. "Keeping quiet just makes it harder for everyone." Lee adds that only by raising awareness of IBS as a real illness that affects millions will there be progress toward greater understanding of the disorder. She writes: "You need a massive amount of strength to cope with IBS. If we all start talking about our symptoms, maybe one day the world will understand that."[44]

> **"Depending on whether people have Crohn's disease or ulcerative colitis, symptoms range from persistent diarrhea and severe abdominal cramps to rectal bleeding, nausea, constipation, and painful bowel movements."**

Tough to Cope

All types of bowel disorders can be difficult for sufferers, and some of the worst are inflammatory bowel diseases. Depending on whether people have Crohn's disease or ulcerative colitis, they may experience symptoms that range from persistent diarrhea and severe abdominal cramps to rectal bleeding, nausea, constipation, and painful bowel movements. Also characteristic of these disorders are psychological problems such as depression and feelings of isolation, as Alexander Noyes explains: "It's really easy to feel alone in your battle and in your struggle with it."[45]

Like Noyes, Janice Chavkin suffers from Crohn's disease, which developed when she was a teenager. At the time of her diagnosis the main treatment prescribed by doctors was steroids, and these medications often caused side effects such as weight gain, acne, and mood swings. Chavkin was affected by these symptoms while also suffering from shame and embarrassment, as she explains: "I became very withdrawn at school and stopped speaking to everybody because I was embarrassed by what I had."[46] By the time she was in college, Chavkin's symptoms had gotten worse. It was not uncommon for her to rush out of class to the bathroom and stay in there for so long that she did not feel comfortable returning to the classroom. When this started happening as often as four times a day, her grades dropped and her embarrassment grew worse.

When Chavkin participated in a clinical trial for a drug called Remicade, she noticed a remarkable improvement in the way she felt. There were risks involved, however, one of which was an increased chance of developing cancer—and ten years after starting the treatment, she was diagnosed with cancer of the cervix. Chavkin underwent a complete hysterectomy and has remained cancer free ever since, although she is the first to say that Crohn's disease has profoundly affected her life. Her doctor said that no matter what the disease did to her, she must not let it stop her from doing what she needed or wanted to do, and Chavkin has worked hard at taking that advice to heart. "If I wanted to," she says, "I could sit around and mope and cry all day, but I'm not going to let it get there."[47]

"Suffering from heartburn on a regular basis can be miserable—and it can also be risky."

The Misery of GERD

Suffering from heartburn on a regular basis can be miserable—and it can also be risky. When the lower esophageal sphincter is not functioning normally, it can result in a constant backwash of acid that irritates the lining of the esophagus and causes it to become chronically inflamed. According to the Mayo Clinic, this inflammation can lead to serious complications such as a narrowing of the esophagus, known as esophageal stricture: "Damage to cells in the lower esophagus from acid exposure leads to the formation of scar tissue. The scar tissue narrows the food pathway, causing difficulty swallowing."[48]

When Isaac Kassin was in the throes of GERD, his suffering was unbearable at times. "I continued to get very bad heartburn," he says, "and it began to take over my life." He writes:

> I was constantly worried about getting that familiar sour pain, and I began to think about it every second of every day. I woke up worried about it, and slept worried about it. School anxiety, everyday stress, mistakes in dieting, and constant thought of heartburn, did bring on the harsh heartburn. Eventually I convinced myself the dieting and strictness weren't working, and the constant pain began to cause me to lose my mind.[49]

The longer Kassin continued to suffer from severe heartburn, the more his anxiety grew. He began to panic about the possibility of developing cancer or ulcers, as well as about the likelihood that he was going to die. He writes: "I thought I felt lumps in my throat and stomach, and that every tiny sense of pain was deathly. I began to spiral out of control, and before I knew it, I was in a constant state of worry and depression."[50]

GERD's Deadly Cousin

Many people who suffer from chronic acid reflux have no idea that they are at risk of developing Barrett's esophagus, a condition in which the cells of the lower esophagus become damaged from repeated exposure to stomach acid. According to the NIDDK, anyone can develop the condition (including people who do not have GERD), but it is up to five times more common among those who do suffer from GERD. The American Society for Gastrointestinal Endoscopy adds that Barrett's esophagus is most likely to develop in patients who either experienced GERD first at a young age or have had a longer duration of symptoms.

Barrett's esophagus is a condition that must be closely monitored because it increases the risk for developing a kind of cancer called esophageal adenocarcinoma. This is a vicious and aggressive form of cancer that has a five-year survival rate of less than 15 percent. The good news is that esophageal adenocarcinoma is extremely rare, affecting only about one in two hundred people with Barrett's esophagus. The not-so-good news is that experts say adenocarcinoma's prevalence is on the rise; in fact, it is often deemed the fastest growing cancer in the United States. Although numbers vary from source to source, studies have shown that there has been at least a 400 percent increase in esophageal adenocarcinoma since the 1970s. New York City physician Jonathan LaPook offers a possible reason why: "The obesity epidemic may well be playing a role by increasing the number of adults with acid reflux."[51]

A Life-Threatening Situation

According to Jay W. Marks, a gastroenterologist in Mission Viejo, California, most people who develop peptic ulcers "generally function quite comfortably." Many complications are possible, however, one of which is bleeding. When someone has a bleeding ulcer, this can lead to overall weakness, the vomiting of blood, dizziness, and fainting. Immediate treatment is essential, as Marks explains: "Initial treatment involves rapid replacement of lost blood intravenously, usually with fluids. Patients with persistent or severe bleeding may require blood transfusions."[52] In April 2011 fourteen-year-old Stephen Cohn from Buffalo Grove, Illinois, was found to have two bleeding ulcers while on a spring break Caribbean cruise with his parents—and he came perilously close to dying.

> **Barrett's esophagus is a condition that must be closely monitored because it increases the risk for developing a kind of cancer called esophageal adenocarcinoma.**

Cohn's problem started on a sunny day at sea when he was hanging out with some other kids at a cruise ship youth program. Seemingly out of nowhere he felt sick, so he went back to his room, and before long he was vomiting blood. He called for help, and a crew member ran to his aid and phoned the ship's emergency 911 line. Cohn was taken to an onboard clinic where medical staff determined that he had lost an extensive amount of blood. When his vomiting resumed, and he again passed out, the captain contacted the US Coast Guard, which sent a helicopter to meet the ship. In the middle of the night, strapped into a harness, Cohn was lifted into the helicopter and flown along with his mother and a cruise ship nurse to a hospital in Rio Piedras, Puerto Rico, where he received emergency care. Cohn recovered completely, and today he does not remember much about his close brush with death. "I was looking forward to a weeklong cruise and some stories to tell about spring break," he says. "But this is one heckuva story."[53]

When Gluten Is the Enemy

It is essential for people with celiac disease to avoid eating anything that contains gluten. This is true not only because they can have a flare-up of painful symptoms but also because of the potential damage the disease can inflict on their bodies. For example, the small intestine is lined with millions of microscopic villi whose function is to absorb vitamins, minerals, and other nutrients that the body needs to stay healthy. When people with celiac disease eat gluten, an immune system reaction to the protein causes damage to the villi so they can no longer absorb essential nutrients. Mayo Clinic gastroenterologist Joseph A. Murray compares normal villi to thick, deep-pile carpet, whereas in someone with untreated celiac disease, the intestine "looks like a tile floor."[54]

> **One of the most serious long-term risks posed by the malnourishment of celiac disease is osteoporosis, a condition in which the bones lose density and become brittle and more likely to fracture.**

Young people with celiac disease are at risk of not growing properly and may suffer from anemia (an insufficient number of healthy red blood cells), abnormal weight loss, and chronic fatigue. They may also bruise easily, have muscle cramps and joint pain, and suffer from nosebleeds. One of the most serious long-term risks posed by the malnourishment of celiac disease is osteoporosis, a condition in which the bones lose density and become brittle and more likely to fracture. According to the National Institutes of Health (NIH), more than 40 million people in the United States suffer from osteoporosis or are at high risk for developing it. The NIH writes: "It has been called a childhood disease with old age consequences because building healthy bones in youth helps prevent osteoporosis and fractures later in life."[55]

A study published in July 2011 focused on evaluating the risk of osteoporosis among celiac disease sufferers. Researchers from the Lancaster University School of Health and Medicine in the United Kingdom took bone density readings of approximately one thousand adults with celiac disease. They found that the risk of developing osteoporosis is four times higher among people who suffer from celiac disease than among the general population.

"A Unique Group"

From the chronic diarrhea and severe abdominal pain that are characteristic of irritable bowel syndrome to the miserable heartburn of GERD and long-term risks of celiac disease, digestive disorders can wreak havoc on people's quality of life. Kassin is an example of someone who has suffered a great deal because of both GERD and celiac disease, and who has struggled with emotional pain because of it. Yet despite some tough times over the years, he embraces life, remains positive, and uses his experience to be a better person and help others. "The pain has allowed me to open my heart to others," says Kassin. "I have developed an ability to feel and sympathize with people's pains and discomforts. When one describes an emotional or physical distress, I immediately feel the ache the person is referring to. I feel lucky to have developed this gift because I feel like an exclusive member to a unique group."[56]

Primary Source Quotes*

What Are the Effects of Digestive Disorders?

"While some digestive diseases are common and others quite rare, collectively, they exact a significant toll on public health in terms of their effects on quality of life, years lost due to premature death, and costs associated with hospitalization and pharmaceutical and surgical interventions."

National Institute of Diabetes and Digestive and Kidney Diseases (NIDDK), *Digestive Diseases and Nutrition*, February 2011. www2.niddk.nih.gov.

The NIDDK conducts and supports medical research and research training to improve the health and quality of life of people suffering from diabetes and digestive and kidney diseases.

"From a child's perspective, one of the most upsetting effects of inflammatory bowel disease is its suppression of growth and sexual maturity."

American Academy of Pediatrics, "Irritable Bowel Syndrome (IBS) and Inflammatory Bowel Disease (IBD)," Healthy Children, January 6, 2012. www.healthychildren.org.

The American Academy of Pediatrics is dedicated to the health, safety, and well-being of infants, children, adolescents, and young adults.

* Editor's Note: While the definition of a primary source can be narrowly or broadly defined, for the purposes of Compact Research, a primary source consists of: 1) results of original research presented by an organization or researcher; 2) eyewitness accounts of events, personal experience, or work experience; 3) first-person editorials offering pundits' opinions; 4) government officials presenting political plans and/or policies, 5) representatives of organizations presenting testimony or policy.

"Living with digestive health problems can be challenging. Digestive health problems can impact on your ability to enjoy foods and beverages, can affect your ability to work and engage in social situations, can limit personal relationships, and can decrease quality of life."

Raymond Cross, "Avoiding Digestive Health Problems," University of Maryland Medical Center, February 4, 2010. www.umm.edu.

Cross is director of the University of Maryland Medical Center's Inflammatory Bowel Disease Program and codirector of the Digestive Health Center.

"Contracting a chronic illness such as Crohn's is a life-changing event."

John Bradley, *The Foul Bowel: 101 Ways to Survive and Thrive with Crohn's Disease*. Oakville, ON: Yknot, 2010, p. 117.

Bradley is an author and former marketing executive who has battled Crohn's disease since he was in his twenties.

"When GERD is not treated, serious complications can occur, such as severe chest pain that can mimic a heart attack, esophageal stricture (a narrowing or obstruction of the esophagus), bleeding, or a pre-malignant change in the lining of the esophagus called Barrett's esophagus."

American College of Gastroenterology, "Acid Reflux," 2012. http://patients.gi.org.

Composed of more than twelve thousand physicians, the American College of Gastroenterology seeks to advance the medical treatment and scientific study of gastrointestinal disorders.

"Over time, untreated ulcers grow larger and deeper and can lead to other problems, such as bleeding in the digestive system or a hole in the wall of the stomach or duodenum, which can make someone very sick."

American Academy of Family Physicians, "Ulcers," September 2012. http://kidshealth.org.

The American Academy of Family Physicians represents more than one hundred thousand family physicians, medical residents, and medical students.

“Children and adults with untreated celiac disease may become malnourished, meaning they do not get enough nutrients, resulting in anemia, weight loss, and, in children, delayed growth and small stature.”

National Institutes of Health (NIH), “What People with Celiac Disease Need to Know About Osteoporosis,” January 2012. www.niams.nih.gov.

The NIH is an agency of the US Department of Health and Human Services and the largest source of medical research funding in the world.

“Until recently an increased risk of cancer was thought to exist mainly for ulcerative colitis patients, but it is now known that Crohn’s patients have an increased risk of colon cancer as well.”

Centers for Disease Control and Prevention (CDC), “Inflammatory Bowel Disease,” May 1, 2012. www.cdc.gov.

The CDC is a federal agency dedicated to protecting health and promoting quality of life through the prevention and control of disease, injury, and disability.

“Peptic ulcers can eat a hole through the wall of your stomach or small intestine, putting you at risk of serious infection of your abdominal cavity.”

Mayo Clinic, “Peptic Ulcer,” January 6, 2011. www.mayoclinic.com.

The Mayo Clinic is a world-renowned medical facility headquartered in Rochester, Minnesota.

Facts and Illustrations

What Are the Effects of Digestive Disorders?

- According to the American College of Gastroenterology, when gastroesophageal reflux disease (GERD) remains untreated, the reflux of acids into the esophagus can damage its lining and lead to **bleeding and scarring**.
- Studies by Mayo Clinic researchers have shown that undiagnosed and untreated **celiac disease** can quadruple the risk of death.
- According to the Children's Hospital of Wisconsin, long-term digestive disorder problems can deplete important nutrients in children, causing **malnutrition** that affects their physical and mental growth and development.
- The University of Maryland Medical Center states that up to **60 percent** of people with irritable bowel syndrome have psychological problems such as anxiety and depression.
- According to pediatrician Andrew B. Grossman, people with Crohn's disease often are **undernourished** due to poor appetite, avoidance of eating due to pain or discomfort, and/or poor absorption of nutrients by the damaged intestines.
- The National Institute of Diabetes and Digestive and Kidney Diseases states that ulcerative colitis can cause problems such as **joint pain, eye irritation, kidney stones, and liver disease**.

IBS Impairs Quality of Life

People who suffer from irritable bowel syndrome (IBS) say it interferes with their daily lives. To evaluate the impact of IBS on quality of life, a team of researchers from Singapore conducted a study that was published in August 2012. The study found that people with IBS suffer from higher levels of physical pain and psychological distress than non-sufferers.

Health-related quality of life: IBS sufferers versus non-sufferers

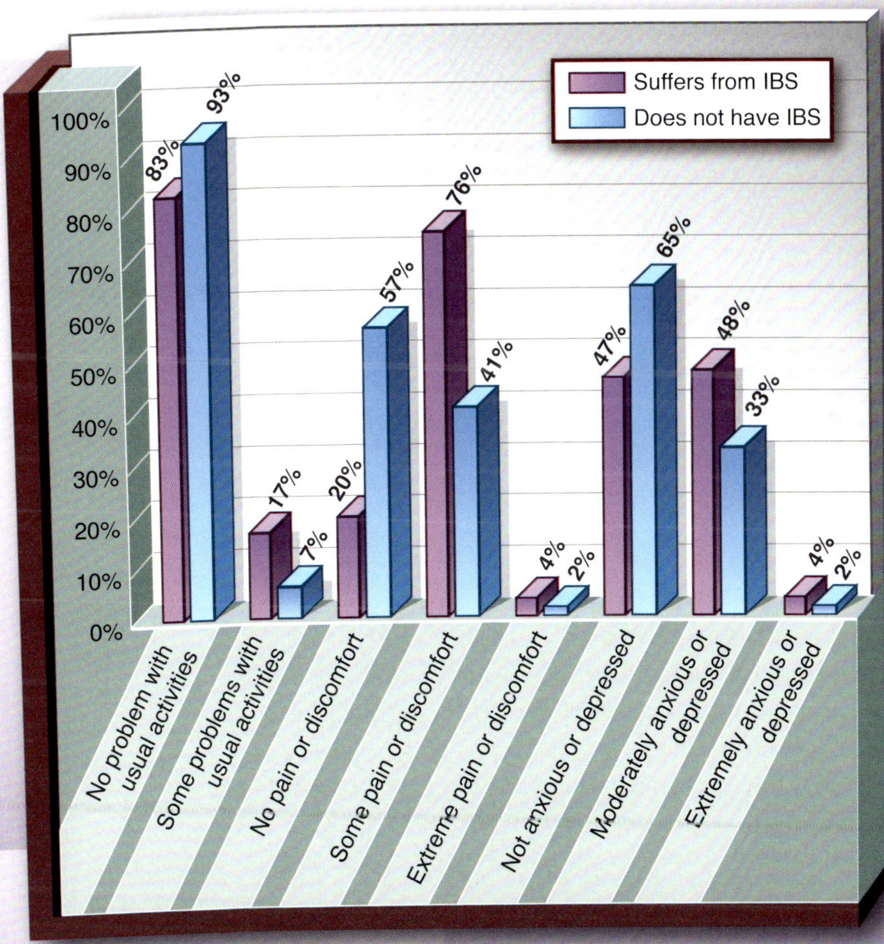

Source: Yu Tien Wang et al., "The Impact of Irritable Bowel Syndrome on Health-Related Quality of Life: A Singapore Perspective," *BMC Gastroenterology*, August 9, 2012. www.biomedcentral.com.

A High-Risk Digestive Disease

For people with celiac disease, keeping gluten out of their diets is essential. Those who do not follow a strict gluten-free diet risk developing life-threatening complications.

Potential complications of untreated celiac disease
Autoimmune disorders (in which the immune system functions abnormally)
Bone disease (such as osteoporosis)
Certain types of intestinal cancer
Anemia (deficiency of red blood cells)
Hypoglycemia (low blood sugar)
Infertility or repeated miscarriage
Liver disease

Source: UPMC Digestive Disorders Center, "Celiac Disease—Sprue," January 20, 2010. www.upmc.com.

- US Navy physician Theodore W. Schafer states that bleeding from an ulcer may be slow and unnoticed or erupt in a **life-threatening hemorrhage**.
- According to the National Institutes of Health, one risk for people who suffer from celiac disease and are not treated is the development of **osteoporosis**, a loss of bone density.
- According to the Mayo Clinic, chronic constipation in children could be caused by **Hirschsprung's disease**, a condition that results from missing nerve cells in the colon.

Bowel Diseases Interfere with Physical Fitness

Many people with Crohn's disease or ulcerative colitis become so discouraged by symptoms like uncontrollable diarrhea, fatigue, and severe pain that they give up trying to participate in exercise and sports. To gain a better understanding of this problem, the British charitable organization Crohn's & Colitis UK conducted a survey and released the findings in May 2012. This graph shows responses when participants were asked why they cut back on or gave up exercise.

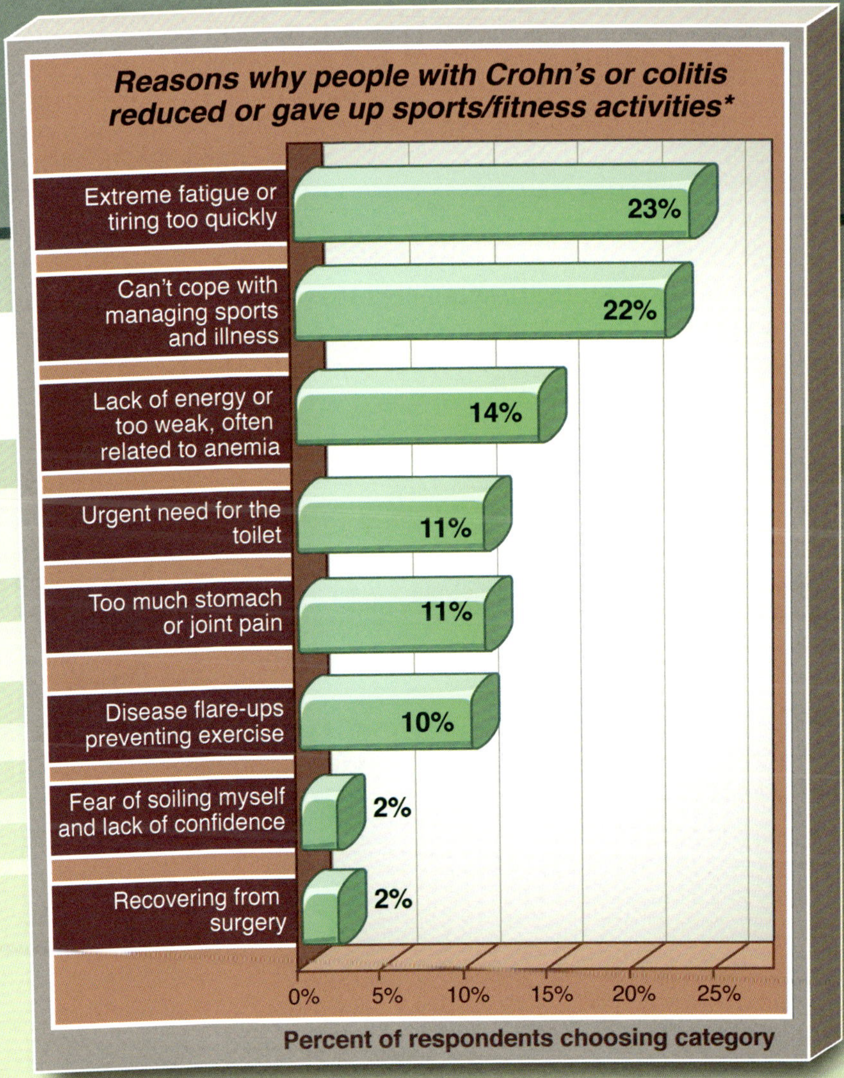

* Shown are the most frequent answer given, so numbers do not total 100 percent.

Source: Crohn's & Colitis UK, "Inflammatory Bowel Disease (IBD) Sport and Fitness Survey Overview and Key Insights," May 2012. www.nacc.org.uk.

How Are Digestive Disorders Treated?

"Digestive diseases can range in severity from troublesome to life-threatening. Fortunately, new advances in research and technology have greatly improved the diagnosis and treatment of these conditions."

H.H. Chao Comprehensive Digestive Disease Center, which is located at the University of California–Irvine and provides specialized care to patients with digestive disorders.

"There are always new treatments and possibilities looming on the horizon."

American College of Gastroenterology, which seeks to advance the medical treatment and scientific study of gastrointestinal disorders.

For more than ten years Adam Vasser kept his chronic acid reflux disease under control by taking proton pump inhibitors, medications that reduce the amount of acid produced by the stomach. In 2010, however, the drugs stopped working for him, and his symptoms returned—with a vengeance. Night was by far the worst time, as Vasser would wake up choking on partially digested food and liquid, his throat burning from stomach acid. Surgery was the obvious choice, but as a teenager Vasser had undergone a heart transplant, and internal scarring made surgery more difficult and risky. So, his doctors recommended that he undergo a new type of procedure that would reconstruct the barrier between the stomach and esophagus. Rather than requiring incisions to be made in Vasser's abdomen, the procedure would be performed through his mouth.

In August 2011 Vasser underwent the operation at Stanford Hospital & Clinics in Palo Alto, California. First, he was given anesthesia, and then surgeons began the procedure using a device known as the EsophyX, which has been likened to a "high-tech fishing pole."[57] The flexible rod was inserted into Vasser's mouth and down his throat until it reached his stomach. Then a tiny retractable wire grabbed a small patch of the stomach wall and pulled it down. The two sides of the resulting flap were pressed together and shaped with the help of a tissue mold, and held in place with plastic fasteners. The process was repeated on adjoining sections of the stomach wall until a semicircular valve was formed just beneath the lower esophagus.

"Physicians typically start by recommending lifestyle changes such as quitting smoking, eating a healthier diet, keeping weight under control, reducing alcohol intake (or avoiding it altogether), and eliminating acid-triggering foods like carbonated beverages, chocolate, and coffee."

The procedure eliminated GERD by tightening Vasser's lower esophageal sphincter and reestablishing a barrier to reflux. Afterward, he was able to leave the hospital in less than twenty-four hours and says it has made an amazing difference in how he feels—as well as in his ability to sleep at night.

Getting Over GERD

Treatments for people with chronic acid reflux vary depending on the severity of their symptoms. Physicians typically start by recommending lifestyle changes such as quitting smoking, eating a healthier diet, keeping weight under control, reducing alcohol intake (or avoiding it altogether), and eliminating acid-triggering foods like carbonated beverages, chocolate, and coffee. Although GERD sufferers often improve after making these changes, what works for one person may not be effective for someone else.

Several types of medications can help relieve GERD symptoms. For example, over-the-counter antacids (Alka-Seltzer or Maalox) work by neutralizing stomach acid and can often help with mild heartburn. Stronger medications called H_2 blockers are so-named because they block histamine, which stimulates the secretion of stomach acid. Proton pump inhibitors work by halting the mechanism that pumps acid into the stomach. Some of these are also available over-the-counter, whereas others must be prescribed by a physician. A class of medications called prokinetics can also be used to reduce the frequency of acid reflux by strengthening the lower esophageal sphincter muscle, as well as helping the stomach empty faster.

> **Because the most common cause of peptic ulcers is *H. pylori* infection, treatment often consists of antibiotics that kill the bacteria.**

Many GERD sufferers benefit from a combination of medications, as the Nemours Foundation explains: "For example, people who get heartburn after eating can try taking both antacids and H_2 blockers. The antacid goes to work first to neutralize the acid in the stomach, while the H_2 blocker acts on acid production. By the time the antacid stops working, the H_2 blocker will have stopped acid production."[58]

Relief from the LINX

People with especially severe cases of GERD who are not helped by traditional treatment methods may benefit from a new device that was approved for use by the US Food and Drug Administration (FDA) in March 2012. Known as the LINX reflux management system, the device consists of magnetic titanium beads strung on titanium wires. It is surgically placed around the patient's lower esophageal sphincter, where the magnetized beads provide extra force to keep the sphincter closed. As needed, the ring of beads enlarges to allow the passage of food when a patient swallows, and then closes again at the appropriate time.

Prior to the FDA's approval of the LINX device, a clinical study showed it to be effective for people suffering from GERD. Of one hundred patients who were implanted with it, sixty-four either had normal amounts of acid in the esophagus or at least a 50 percent reduction. Additionally, ninety-two of the patients showed marked improvement in their GERD symptoms, and the same amount were able to reduce their medicines or no longer needed to take any medicines to treat their GERD symptoms.

Treatments for Ulcers

Because the most common cause of peptic ulcers is *H. pylori* infection, treatment often consists of antibiotics that kill the bacteria. According to the NIDDK, antibiotic regimens may differ throughout the world since some *H. pylori* strains have become resistant to certain antibiotics, meaning that a drug that was once effective at destroying the bacterium is no longer effective. The group writes: "Doctors closely follow research on antibiotic treatments for *H. pylori* infection to know which treatment strategy will destroy which strain."[59]

> **"People who are newly diagnosed with irritable bowel syndrome are often discouraged to find out that there is no cure, nor are there medications specifically designed to treat it."**

Experts say that antibiotics can cure up to 90 percent of ulcers caused by *H. pylori*, but eliminating the bacteria can be difficult. About a month after treatment begins, patients undergo a breath or stool test so the physician can evaluate whether the infection has been cured. (Blood tests are not used because patients may still test positive for *H. pylori* even after the bacteria have been killed.) According to the NIDDK, if tests show that *H. pylori* is still present, additional antibiotic treatment will be necessary until all the bacteria have been eliminated.

As effective as antibiotics can be, some ulcer sufferers do not respond to the medications. This was the case with a British woman named Freya Pietzsch, who was diagnosed with an ulcer after testing positive for *H. pylori*. "I thought treating it would simply be a matter of a short course of antibiotics to clear it up," she says, "and that is exactly what my GP [general practitioner] gave me. But the symptoms came back again soon after I stopped the antibiotics and I began to get concerned. I hadn't taken it very seriously until I read that ulcers in the stomach could be one of the causes of stomach cancer." Pietzsch's doctor prescribed a different antibiotic, but it caused side effects such as headaches and tingling in her arms and legs, so she stopped taking it. She started to get worried because nothing was working and the ulcer was making her sick. "I didn't know what else I could try,"[60] she says.

Pietzsch happened to hear about a substance called mastic gum, which is a natural resin that comes from pistachio nuts. She was told that the gum cured a friend's ulcer, and after doing some research she ordered the substance in tablet form and began taking it every day. She was astounded that after three weeks her ulcer symptoms had subsided, and they were practically gone within a month. According to Dlawer Al-deen, who is a microbiologist at Nottingham City Hospital in the United Kingdom, mastic gum is far from a new treatment for ulcers. He has conducted his own studies with it, as he explains: "It has been known for many years that mastic gum can help clear up peptic ulcers and there have been several clinical studies on its effects in countries outside the UK in the past decade. But my attention was caught when I realised that mastic gum in higher doses—up to three grams a day—actually killed the H pylori bacteria permanently."[61] Mastic gum is considered an alternative treatment for peptic ulcers, although it is used in other countries much more often than the United States.

The Healing Power of the Mind

People who are newly diagnosed with irritable bowel syndrome are often discouraged to find out that there is no cure, nor are there medications specifically designed to treat it. Doctors typically recommend changes to diet and lifestyle that can help reduce the severity of symptoms. Says psychologist Stephen R. Weinland: "Often, learning to implement good sleep, hygiene, stress reduction, and other coping strategies for dealing with situations can go a long way in making you feel more in control of your symptoms, rather than feeling like IBS is controlling you. Increasing your control over symptoms is another one of the steps towards improvement in your IBS."[62]

In addition to lifestyle changes to help an IBS sufferer, Weinland says physicians often recommend professional therapy. This advice is not always well received, however, as people may interpret this to mean that the doctor thinks they are imagining their symptoms. Says Weinland: "This reaction often comes from the belief that a referral to a psychologist carries with it assumptions about symptoms being 'all in your head' or the result of 'mental illness.' These are two of the biggest misconceptions about the practice of psychology in a medical setting, and they can often stand in the way of patients achieving a meaningful reduction in symptoms."[63]

> **"Crohn's disease sufferers can do themselves a world of good by eating right, taking the prescribed medications, and doing everything possible to avoid flare-ups."**

Weinland says that psychologists and physicians work as a team with the understanding that the mind and body are connected. "If you are feeling ill and having many symptoms of IBS," he says, "you may also experience an increased level of stress and discomfort. This stress and discomfort contribute to a cycle of worsening symptoms that can spiral into more severe IBS. Psychologists and physicians work together with you to interrupt that cycle and help you learn to decrease the number and severity of your symptoms."[64]

The Value of Meditation

As with many diseases and disorders, meditation has been shown to help people who suffer from IBS. A study published in 2011 showed the success of a meditative technique known as mindfulness meditation, which involves focusing on present-moment experience and a nonjudgmental awareness of body sensations and emotions—simply being "in the now." The study involved seventy-five women between the ages of nineteen and seventy-one. Those who were placed in a mindfulness meditation group participated in daily practices and readings, sitting and walking meditation, and yoga. The women in the second group participated in weekly discussions on various topics, readings, and a half-day social retreat.

At the end of the study, symptom severity was reduced in 26.4 percent of the meditation group compared with 6.2 percent of the control group. Says clinical psychologist Olafur S. Palsson, one of the researchers involved in the study: "Our study indicates that mindfulness meditation is a practical, widely applicable and inexpensive method to enable irritable bowel syndrome patients to improve their clinical outcomes and gain associated improvement in well-being."[65] Although mindfulness meditation has proved to be effective, Palsson says that exactly how and why it works is not known, and more research is planned to investigate this.

Help for Crohn's Sufferers

After someone has been diagnosed with Crohn's disease, one of the first recommendations is lifestyle changes, and diet is an important part of that. The foods that sufferers eat can have a major impact on how they feel, and designing the right diet is often a matter of trial and error. Alexander Noyes kept a food journal, which helped him discover that his digestive system was irritated by dairy products and excessive fiber. He limits those foods and eats a diet that revolves around nutrient-dense foods, which he says has given him more energy and helped him feel better overall.

Crohn's disease sufferers can greatly help themselves by eating right, taking the prescribed medications, and doing everything possible to avoid flare-ups. Juliana Santos, a college student who was diagnosed with Crohn's when she was eleven years old, has become an expert at managing her disease. She takes more than twenty pills each day and has changed her diet, meticulously paying attention to every morsel of food she puts in her mouth. For instance, she loves strawberries but cannot eat them because the tiny seeds are difficult for her to digest. Another of her favorites is spicy foods, but she avoids them because of the excruciating pain she will suffer after eating them.

Like anyone with inflammatory bowel disease, Santos has had many challenges along the way and more than her share of suffering. She refuses to let the disease defeat her, however, and wants to be an inspiration for other young people who suffer from it. "I tell them to never stop fighting," she says. "The battle is hard—there's no doubt about that. However, there is still hope."[66]

Hope for the Future

Today, people with digestive disorders have more hope than ever before. Even if they have an illness for which there is no cure, a wide variety of medications and surgical techniques can help relieve symptoms immensely and improve their quality of life. As scientists continue to pursue research, even better treatments will undoubtedly become available, meaning that fewer people will have to suffer from these disorders in the future.

Primary Source Quotes*

How Are Digestive Disorders Treated?

"Fortunately, effective medical treatments usually control most digestive health problems."

Raymond Cross, "Avoiding Digestive Health Problems," University of Maryland Medical Center, February 4, 2010. www.umm.edu.

Cross is director of the University of Maryland Medical Center's Inflammatory Bowel Disease Program and codirector of the Digestive Health Center.

"Several studies of hypnotherapy for IBS have shown substantial long-term improvement of gastrointestinal symptoms as well as anxiety, depression, disability, and quality of life."

National Center for Complementary and Alternative Medicine (NCCAM), "Irritable Bowel Syndrome and CAM: What the Science Says," May 2011. http://nccam.nih.gov.

The NCCAM uses scientific research to investigate the usefulness and safety of complementary and alternative medical treatments in improving health and health care.

---

* Editor's Note: While the definition of a primary source can be narrowly or broadly defined, for the purposes of Compact Research, a primary source consists of: 1) results of original research presented by an organization or researcher; 2) eyewitness accounts of events, personal experience, or work experience; 3) first-person editorials offering pundits' opinions; 4) government officials presenting political plans and/or policies; 5) representatives of organizations presenting testimony or policy.

“The most common medications used to treat digestive disease, proton pump inhibitors, are among the best-selling drugs worldwide, but we are becoming increasingly aware that they produce myriad health problems and are far from a home run as therapy.”

Andrew Weil, foreword to *The Inside Tract: Your Good Gut Guide to Great Digestive Health* by Gerald E. Mullin and Kathie Madonna Swift. New York: Rodale, 2011, p. x.

Weil is well known for being a pioneer in the field of integrative medicine, a holistic approach to health care that encompasses treating body, mind, and spirit.

“Year after year, medications for digestive illness top the pharmaceutical bestseller list.”

Elizabeth Lipski, *Digestive Wellness*. New York: McGraw-Hill, 2012, p. 4.

Lipski is a clinical nutritionist who is director of doctoral studies at Hawthorn University.

“Early effective interventions in children have the potential to prevent or reduce the incidence and/or severity of later functional GI disorders in adults.”

International Foundation for Functional Gastrointestinal Disorders (IFFGD), “Kids & Teens,” August 22, 2012. www.iffgd.org.

The IFFGD is an educational and research organization that seeks to inform, assist, and support people who are affected by gastrointestinal disorders.

“Irritable bowel syndrome (IBS) is often treated with alternative therapies. Stress reduction techniques, such as biofeedback, hypnosis, dietary changes, or counseling, may help.”

University of Maryland Medical Center, “Irritable Bowel Syndrome,” January 20, 2012. www.umm.edu.

The University of Maryland Medical Center is a teaching hospital in Baltimore, Maryland.

“Surgery becomes necessary in Crohn’s disease when medications can no longer control the symptoms.”

Centers for Disease Control and Prevention (CDC), “Inflammatory Bowel Disease,” May 1, 2012. www.cdc.gov.

The CDC is a federal agency dedicated to protecting health and promoting quality of life through the prevention and control of disease, injury, and disability.

“Numerous homeopathic remedies exist for constipation, and they typically consist of plant-based laxatives. However, just because they’re natural doesn’t mean they’re safe.”

Mayo Clinic, “Constipation,” January 14, 2011. www.mayoclinic.com.

The Mayo Clinic is a world-renowned medical facility headquartered in Rochester, Minnesota.

“People used to believe drinking milk helped peptic ulcers heal. But doctors know now that while milk may make an ulcer feel better briefly, it also increases stomach acid, which can make ulcers worse.”

The National Institute of Diabetes and Digestive and Kidney Diseases (NIDDK), “*H. Pylori* and Peptic Ulcers,” April 30, 2012. http://digestive.niddk.nih.gov.

The NIDDK conducts and supports medical research and research training to improve the health and quality of life of people suffering from diabetes and digestive and kidney diseases.

“The only treatment for celiac disease is to follow a gluten-free diet.”

National Institutes of Health (NIH), “What People with Celiac Disease Need to Know About Osteoporosis,” January 2012. www.niams.nih.gov.

The NIH is an agency of the US Department of Health and Human Services and the largest source of medical research funding in the world.

How Are Digestive Disorders Treated?

- According to New York dietician Tamara Duker Freuman, drugs known as **proton pump inhibitors** are the most common medications prescribed for people with acid reflux.

- The Mayo Clinic states that most cases of constipation can be resolved with simple **changes in diet and lifestyle**.

- According to Johns Hopkins Medicine, up to **90 percent** of people with peptic ulcers caused by *Helicobacter pylori* bacteria can be permanently cured with antibiotics treatment.

- A report release in August 2012 by Mayo Clinic researchers states that of the estimated 1.8 million Americans with celiac disease, roughly **80 percent** are never diagnosed or treated.

- The National Institute of Diabetes and Digestive and Kidney Diseases states that surgery may be the best option for children with severe **gastroesophageal reflux disease (GERD)** if symptoms do not respond to medication.

- In October 2012 researchers announced that a drug called **Stelara**, which is used to treat the skin disorder psoriasis, showed promising results for people with severe Crohn's disease.

Options for Ulcer Sufferers

Treatment for peptic ulcers depends on whether a patient is infected with the *Helicobacter pylori* bacterium, or has developed the ulcer due to other factors. The goal of treatment is to relieve pain, heal the ulcer, and prevent complications.

Treatment	Purpose/Expected outcome
Antibiotics	Kill the *H. pylori* bacterium, so medications are only recommended for those who are infected by it
Proton pump inhibitor medications	Reduce acid by blocking the action of the parts of cells that produce it, thus promoting healing
Histamine (H_2) blocker medications	Reduce the amount of acid released into the digestive tract, which relieves pain and encourages healing
Antacids	Neutralize stomach acid and can provide rapid pain relief
Cytoprotective medications	Protect the tissues that line the stomach and small intestine

Source: Mayo Clinic, "Peptic Ulcer," January 6, 2011. www.mayoclinic.com.

- The American College of Gastroenterology states that treatment goals for **GERD** are to eliminate symptoms, heal the esophagus, and prevent relapse.

- US Navy physician Theodore W. Schafer states that people being treated for **ulcers** do not need to follow a specific diet.

- According to the American College of Gastroenterology, most cases of **acute diarrhea** can be resolved quickly, without antibiotic therapy, by implementing simple dietary modifications.

Implant Reduces GERD Symptoms

Many people who suffer from gastroesophageal reflux disease (GERD) can overcome the condition by taking medications that reduce acid production in the digestive tract. But for some of those with treatment-resistant forms of GERD, a new procedure called the LINX Reflux Management System is being tried. It consists of a ring of titanium beads surgically implanted around the esophagus to help the lower esophageal sphincter perform better. This illustration shows the LINX device and how it works.

LINX device consists of a series of titanium beads connected into a ring with titanium wires.

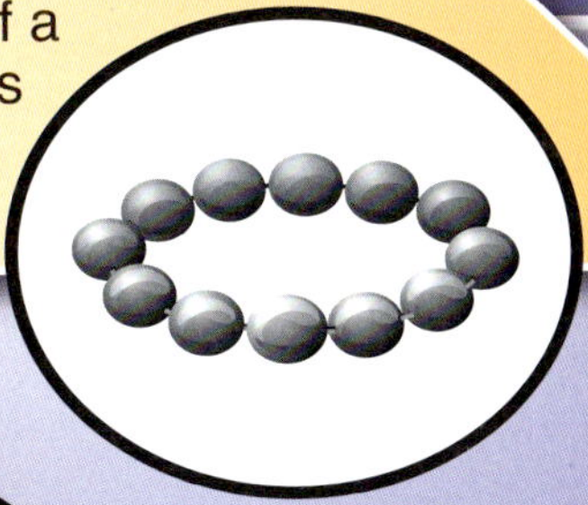

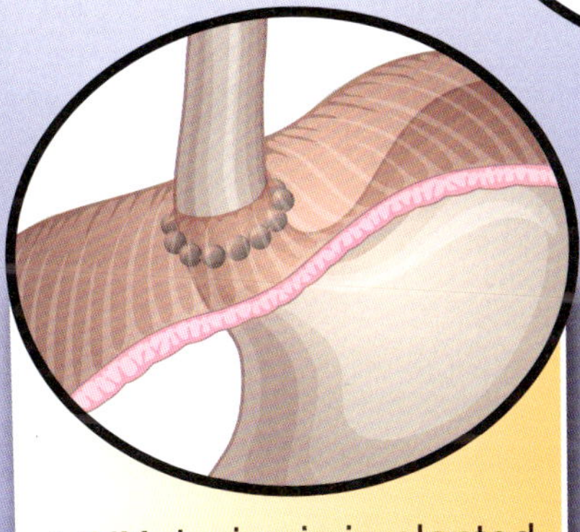

LINX device is implanted around the lower esophageal sphincter.

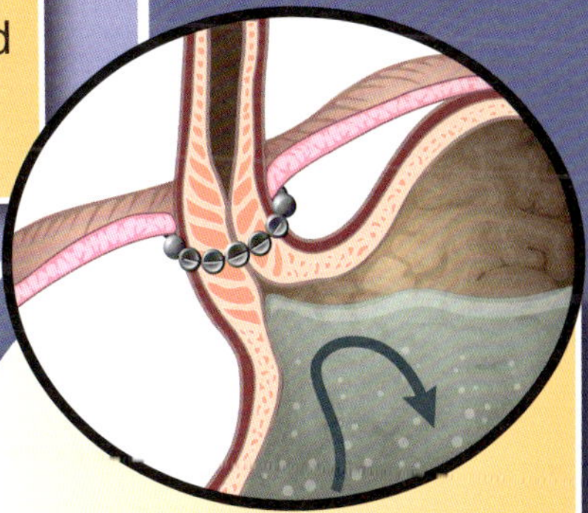

LINX device restricts the flow of stored contents from backing up (refluxing) into the esophagus.

Source: US Food and Drug Administration, "LINX Reflux Management System—P100049," March 22, 2012. www.fda.gov.

The Healing Effects of Meditation

Meditation can help control the symptoms of irritable bowel syndrome (IBS), according to a study published in September 2011. The study looked at two groups. One group practiced mindfulness meditation therapy—which involves focusing on present-moment experience and awareness of body sensations and emotions—and did self-help readings, sitting and walking meditation, and yoga. The other group (a social-support group) gathered for shared meals and discussions on various topics and did self-help readings but did not do meditation. This graph shows the progress of the two groups.

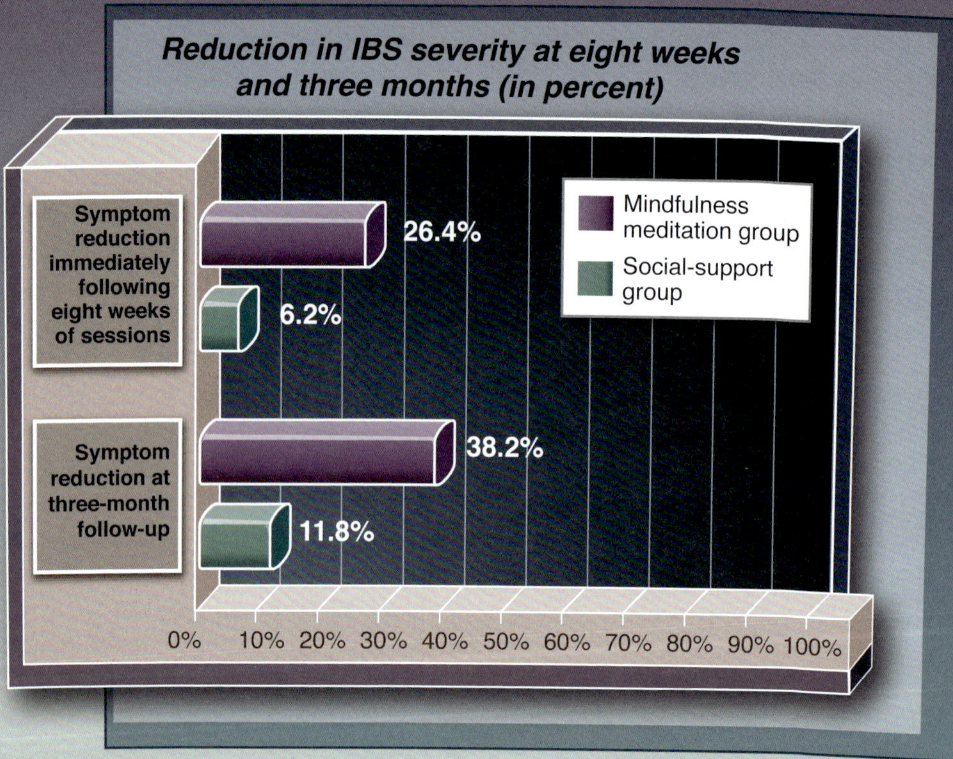

Source: National Center for Complementary and Alternative Medicine, "Mindfulness Meditation Reduces Severity of IBS in Women, Study Finds," March 19, 2012. http://nccam.nih.gov.

- According to the Centers for Disease Control and Prevention (CDC), over the long term, up to **75 percent** of patients with Crohn's disease and **25 percent** of those with ulcerative colitis will require surgery.

- The Mayo Clinic states that in some peptic ulcer cases, doctors prescribe medications called **cytoprotective agents**, which help protect the tissues that line the stomach and small intestine.

- The National Institutes of Health states that a small percentage of people with celiac disease do not improve on a gluten-free diet and may need to receive **intravenous nutrition supplements**.

- According to research presented at the 2011 meeting of the American College of Gastroenterology, at least one-quarter of heartburn sufferers who take drugs known as **proton pump inhibitors** do not need them and are putting their health at risk by taking the drugs unnecessarily.

Key People and Advocacy Groups

American College of Gastroenterology: An organization devoted to advancing the medical treatment and scientific study of gastrointestinal disorders.

Norman Barrett: A British surgeon who, in 1950, described a severe acid reflux disorder that later became known as Barrett's esophagus, a precursor to esophageal cancer.

William Beaumont: An American surgeon who was the first to observe the process of digestion as it occurs in the human stomach, and who became known as the father of gastric physiology.

Burrill B. Crohn: An American gastroenterologist known for his studies of ileitis, an inflammation of the lower small intestine. Crohn's disease, one of the main types of inflammatory bowel disease, was named after him.

Crohn's & Colitis Foundation of America: A volunteer-driven organization that is dedicated to finding cures for inflammatory bowel diseases.

Willem-Karel Dicke: A Dutch pediatrician who in 1941 was the first to identify gluten intolerance and to develop a gluten-free diet.

Barry J. Marshall: An Australian physician who, along with colleague J. Robin Warren, discovered that a type of bacteria called *Helicobacter pylori* (*H. pylori*) was responsible for most peptic ulcers.

National Digestive Diseases Information Clearinghouse (NDDIC): The information dissemination service of the National Institute of Diabetes and Digestive and Kidney Diseases.

J. Robin Warren: An Australian pathologist who, along with colleague Barry J. Marshall, discovered the *Helicobacter pylori* (*H. pylori*) bacteria responsible for most peptic ulcers.

Chronology

1807
German army surgeon Philipp Bozzini invents an instrument he calls the *Lichtleiter* (light guide) to enable him to locate bullets inside wounded soldiers' bodies. Although clumsy and difficult to use, the device proves to be the precursor to the modern endoscope.

1875
British physicians Samuel S. Wilks and Walter Moxon are the first to describe the inflammatory bowel disease known as ulcerative colitis and to differentiate it from diarrhea caused by infectious bacteria.

1887
During a lecture in London, British pediatrician Samuel Gee attributes chronic indigestion (now known to be associated with celiac disease) to "errors in diet," but he does not know which dietary problems are involved.

1908
American physician Christian Archibald Herter publishes a book in which he describes what he calls "intestinal infantilism," a digestive disorder that involves gluten intolerance.

1800 1900 1930 1960

1932
American gastroenterologist Burrill B. Crohn and colleagues Leon Ginzburg and Gordon D. Oppenheimer publish a paper titled "Regional Ileitis: A Pathologic and Chronic Entity," which describes chronic inflammation of the intestinal tract that is later named Crohn's disease.

1941
Dutch pediatrician Willem-Karel Dicke publishes a paper titled "A Simple Diet for Gee-Herter's Syndrome," in which he describes the digestive disorder that later becomes known as celiac disease and explains how it can be treated with a gluten-free diet.

1950
British surgeon Norman Barrett publishes an article in which he describes a severe acid reflux disorder that later becomes known as Barrett's esophagus, a precursor to esophageal cancer.

1958
World Gastroenterology Organization secretary-general Henry Cohen declares May 29 to be World Digestive Health Day, which is intended to increase public awareness of digestive disorder prevention and treatment.

1976
The US Congress establishes the Commission on Digestive Diseases Research, which is charged with determining the prevalence of digestive diseases in the United States, as well as what treatments are available.

2011
A study by researchers in Milan, Italy, finds that many people who believe they are lactose intolerant actually suffer from psychological issues.

1980

2000

1991
Researchers from the Baylor University College of Medicine in Houston publish the first randomized study in the United States that proves the effectiveness of antibiotics in treating ulcers.

2003
Research by the Centers for Disease Control and Prevention finds that the majority of Americans still mistakenly believe that peptic ulcers are caused by stress.

2005
Australian physicians Barry J. Marshall and J. Robin Warren are awarded the Nobel Prize for Medicine or Physiology for their discovery of *Helicobacter pylori* and its role in the development of peptic ulcers.

2012
In one of the largest genetic studies ever conducted, an international team of scientists identifies over seventy genomic regions associated with inflammatory bowel disease.

Related Organizations

Academy of Nutrition and Dietetics

120 S. Riverside Plaza, Suite 2000
Chicago, IL 60606-6995
phone: (312) 899-0040; toll-free: (800) 877-1600
website: www.eatright.org

The Academy of Nutrition and Dietetics seeks to improve Americans' health and advance the profession of dietetics through research, education, and advocacy. Its website search engine produces articles about irritable bowel syndrome, celiac disease, and other digestive disorders.

American Celiac Disease Alliance

2504 Duxbury Pl.
Alexandria, VA 22308
phone: (703) 622-3331
e-mail: info@americanceliac.org • website: www.americanceliac.org

The American Celiac Disease Alliance represents and advocates on behalf of patients, physicians, researchers, food manufacturers, and other service providers. Its website offers a variety of articles and publications about celiac disease, including what it is, what causes it, and how sufferers can manage the illness.

American College of Gastroenterology

6400 Goldsboro Rd., Suite 200
Bethesda, MD 20817
phone: (301) 263-9000
website: http://patients.gi.org

Composed of more than twelve thousand physicians, the American College of Gastroenterology seeks to advance the medical treatment and scientific study of gastrointestinal disorders. Its website offers videos, podcasts, brochures, fact sheets arranged by topic, and a search engine that produces numerous articles about digestive disorders.

Association of Gastrointestinal Motility Disorders (AGMD)

12 Roberts Dr.
Bedford, MA 01730
phone: (781) 275-1300 • fax: (781) 275-1304
e-mail: digestive.motility@gmail.com
website: www.agmd-gimotility.org

The AGMD serves as an educational resource about digestive motility diseases and disorders for the public and members of the medical and scientific communities. Its website offers numerous fact sheets, brochures, and audiovisual materials that address digestive disorders.

Crohn's & Colitis Foundation of America (CCFA)

386 Park Ave. South, 17th Fl.
New York, NY 10016
phone: (800) 932-2423 • fax: (212) 779-4098
e-mail: info@ccfa.org • website: www.ccfa.org

The CCFA is a volunteer-driven organization that is dedicated to finding cures for the inflammatory bowel diseases Crohn's disease and ulcerative colitis. Its website offers numerous publications about these diseases, including information about what they are; their diagnosis, treatment, and prognosis; and current research findings.

Celiac Disease Foundation

20350 Ventura Blvd., Suite 240
Woodland Hills, CA 91364
phone: (818) 716-1513 • fax: (818) 267-5577
website: http://celiac.org

The Celiac Disease Foundation focuses on celiac disease education, awareness, advocacy, and support services. Its website offers a wide variety of informative publications about celiac disease for patients, parents, and caregivers.

International Foundation for Functional Gastrointestinal Disorders (IFFGD)

PO Box 170864
Milwaukee, WI 53217-8076
phone: (414) 964-1799; toll-free (888) 964-2001 • fax: (414) 964-7176
e-mail: iffgd@iffgd.org • website: www.iffgd.org

The IFFGD is an education and research organization that seeks to inform, assist, and support people affected by gastrointestinal disorders. Its website features a variety of articles about digestive disorders, personal stories, research and clinical trial updates, and news releases.

Mayo Clinic

200 First St. SW
Rochester, MN 55905
phone: (507) 284-2511 • fax: (507) 284-0161
website: www.mayoclinic.com

The Mayo Clinic is a world-renowned medical facility that is dedicated to patient care, education, and research. Its website search engine produces numerous articles about digestive disorders such as acid reflux, constipation, inflammatory bowel disease, and ulcers, among others.

National Center for Complementary and Alternative Medicine (NCCAM)

9000 Rockville Pike
Bethesda, MD 20892
phone: (888) 644-6226
website: http://nccam.nih.gov

Through scientific research, the NCCAM investigates the usefulness and safety of complementary and alternative medical treatments in improving health and health care. Its website search engine produces numerous articles about digestive disorders and alternative treatments.

National Institute of Diabetes and Digestive and Kidney Diseases (NIDDK)

Bldg. 31, Rm. 9A06, MSC 2560
31 Center Dr.
Bethesda, MD 20892-2560
phone: (301) 496-3583
e-mail: nddic@info.niddk.nih.gov
website: http://digestive.niddk.nih.gov

A branch of the National Institutes of Health, the NIDDK conducts and supports medical research and research training to improve the health and quality of life of people suffering from diabetes and digestive and kidney diseases. Its website links to the National Digestive Diseases Information Clearinghouse, which is its information dissemination service.

For Further Research

Books

John Bradley, *The Foul Bowel: 101 Ways to Survive and Thrive with Crohn's Disease*. Oakville, ON: Yknot, 2010.

George Capaccio, *Digestive Disorders*. Tarrytown, NY: Marshall Cavendish Benchmark, 2011.

Dustin Garth James and Liz Scott, *The Complete Idiot's Guide to Digestive Health*. New York: Alpha, 2010.

Sophie Lee, *Sophie's Story: My 20-Year Battle with Irritable Bowel Syndrome*. Sherman Oaks, CA: Health Point Press, 2011.

Elizabeth Lipski, *Digestive Wellness*. New York: McGraw-Hill, 2012.

Anil Minocha and Christine Adamec, *Encyclopedia of the Digestive System and Digestive Disorders*. New York: Facts On File, 2010.

Alvin Newman, *The Essential IBS Book: Understanding and Managing Irritable Bowel Syndrome and Functional Dyspepsia*. Toronto: Robert Rose, 2011.

Periodicals

Tatiana Boncompagni, "Enzymes Try to Grab the Spotlight," *New York Times*, February 22, 2012.

Current Health Teens, a *Weekly Reader Publication*, "Crohn's Is No Fun, but Humor and Friends Can Help," September 2011.

Kim Erickson, "The Enzyme Factor: Digestive Problems Got You Down? An Enzyme Boost May Be Just What You Need," *Better Nutrition*, September 2011.

Good Health, "Digestion: Your In-Depth Introduction to Common Digestive Problems," December 1, 2010.

Amy Norton, "Mixed Evidence on Acupuncture for Irritable Bowels," *Chicago Tribune*, April 25, 2012.

Bonnie Taub-Dix, "How to Beat 5 Embarrassing Ailments with Your Diet," *U.S. News & World Report*, November 15, 2012.

Vera Tweed, "Digestive Defenders: Pint-Size Probiotics Play a Giant Role in Immune Health," *Better Nutrition*, August 2011.

U.S. News & World Report, "8 Common Digestive Problems and How to End Them," September 6, 2012.

USA Today, "Lactose Intolerance May Sometimes Be in the Head, Not the Gut," May 13, 2011.

Internet Sources

American Academy of Pediatrics, "Irritable Bowel Syndrome (IBS) and Inflammatory Bowel Disease (IBD)," HealthyChildren, January 6, 2012. www.healthychildren.org/English/health-issues/conditions/abdominal/Pages/Irritable-Bowel-Syndrome-IBS-and-Inflammatory-Bowel-Disease-IBD.aspx.

Boston Children's Hospital Young Men's Health, "Lactose Intolerance," September 29, 2011. www.youngmenshealthsite.org/lactose_intolerance.html.

Brenda Goodman, "Do You Need a Gluten-Free Diet? Probably Not," WebMD, August 1, 2012. www.webmd.com/digestive-disorders/celiac-disease/news/20120801/most-on-gluten-free-diet-dont-have-celiac-disease.

Isaac J. Kassin, "First Person on Celiac Disease: How It Shaped My Life," Stewardship Report, November 22, 2012. http://stewardshipreport.com/celiac-disease-how-it-shaped-my-life.

Nemours Foundation, "Gastroesophageal Reflux Disease (GERD)," Teens Health, June 2011. http://kidshealth.org/parent/system/surgical/gerd_reflux.html.

Nemours Foundation, "Ulcers," Teens Health, September 2012. http://kidshealth.org/teen/diseases_conditions/digestive/ulcers.html.

Mikel Theobald, "Young and Living with Crohn's," Everyday Health, June 6, 2012. www.everydayhealth.com/crohns-disease/young-and-living-with-crohns.aspx.

Dennis Thompson, "Chronic Heartburn a Growing Problem in U.S.," HealthDay, January 5, 2012. http://health.usnews.com/health-news/diet-fitness/digestive-disorders/articles/2012/01/05/chronic-heartburn-a-growing-problem-in-us.

Source Notes

Overview

1. Quoted in Stephanie Watson, "6 Common Mistakes When You Have Crohn's Disease," WebMD, September 6, 2011. www.webmd.com/ibd-crohns-disease/cd-biologics-10/cd-mistakes-with-crohns.
2. Quoted in Watson, "6 Common Mistakes When You Have Crohn's Disease."
3. Kenneth S. Saladin, *Anatomy & Physiology*. New York: McGraw-Hill Education, 2010, p. 966.
4. Quoted in Chris Iliades, "What Does Your Digestive System Do?," Everyday Health, 2013. www.everydayhealth.com/health-report/better-digestion/what-does-your-digestive-system-do.aspx.
5. Elizabeth Lipski, *Digestive Wellness*. New York: McGraw-Hill, 2012, p. 4.
6. Quoted in *U.S. News & World Report*, "8 Common Digestive Problems and How to End Them," September 6, 2012. http://health.usnews.com/health-news/articles/2012/09/06/8-common-digestive-problems-and-how-to-end-them.
7. National Institute of Diabetes and Digestive and Kidney Diseases, "Celiac Disease," January 27, 2012. http://digestive.niddk.nih.gov/ddiseases/pubs/celiac.
8. Johns Hopkins Medicine, "Irritable Bowel Syndrome," July 28, 2009. http://health.usnews.com/health-conditions/digestive-disorders/irritable-bowel-syndrome.
9. Centers for Disease Control and Prevention, "Inflammatory Bowel Disease," May 1, 2012. www.cdc.gov/ibd.
10. Mayo Clinic, "Peptic Ulcer," January 6, 2011. www.mayoclinic.com/health/peptic-ulcer/DS00242.
11. Jennifer Killick, "'Ulcerative Colitis Is Painful, Crippling and Humiliating," *Guardian* (Manchester, UK), April 29, 2012. www.guardian.co.uk/lifeandstyle/2012/apr/29/ulcerative-colitis-painful-crippling-humiliating.
12. Children's Hospital Boston Center for Young Women's Health, "Lactose Intolerance," September 29, 2011. www.youngwomenshealth.org/lactose.html.
13. UPMC Digestive Disorders Center, "About Us," 2012. www.upmc.com/Services/gastroenterology/about/Pages/default.aspx.
14. Nicolle, "My Teenage Life with IBS: Advice Needed!," Irritable Bowel Syndrome Self-Help and Support Group, May 15, 2012. www.ibsgroup.org/forums/topic/153425-my-teenage-life-with-ibs-advice-needed.
15. Michael F. Picco, "Acid Reflux and GERD: The Same Thing?," Mayo Clinic, January 12, 2011. www.mayoclinic.com/health/heartburn-gerd/AN00998.

Chapter 1: What Are Digestive Disorders?

16. Alysa Bajenaru, "Gluten Stole My Mojo . . . and I Want It Back!," *Inspired RD* (blog), August 3, 2011. http://inspiredrd.com/2011/08/gluten-stole-my-mojo-and-i-want-it-back.html.
17. Alysa Bajenaru, "It's Official—I have Celiac Disease," *Inspired RD* (blog), August 11, 2011. http://inspiredrd.com/2011/08/its-official-i-have-celiac-disease.html.
18. Alysa Bajenaru, "What Celiac Disease Is Really Like," *Inspired RD* (blog), October 25, 2012. http://inspiredrd.com/2012/10/what-celiac-disease-is-really-like.html.
19. Bajenaru, "What Celiac Disease Is Really Like."
20. Bajenaru, "What Celiac Disease Is Really Like."
21. Quoted in William F. Paveley, "From Aretaeus to Crosby: A History of Coeliac Disease," *British Medical Journal*, December 24–31, 1988. www.ncbi.nlm.nih.gov/pmc/articles/PMC1838854/pdf/bmj00317-0028.pdf.

22. German Institute for Quality and Efficiency in Health Care, "Lactose Intolerance," Informed Health Online, February 2, 2012. www.ncbi.nlm.nih.gov/pubmedhealth/PMH0005145.
23. Sandra, "A Daily Struggle with Lactose Intolerance," GoDairyFree, November 2012. www.godairyfree.org/personal-stories/a-daily-struggle-with-lactose-intolerance.
24. Sandra, "A Daily Struggle with Lactose Intolerance."
25. Quoted in *USA Today*, "Lactose Intolerance May Sometimes Be in the Head, Not the Gut," May 13, 2011. http://yourlife.usatoday.com/fitness-food/diet-nutrition/story/2011/05/Lactose-intolerance-may-sometimes-be-in-the-head-not-the-gut/47157492/1.
26. Quoted in Fiona Macrae and Claire Bates, "Is Lactose Intolerance in the Mind? Poor Diets May Be to Blame for 'Allergy' Boom," *Daily Mail* (London), September 14, 2011. www.dailymail.co.uk/health/article-2036827/Is-lactose-intolerance-mind-Poor-diets-blame-allergy-boom.html.
27. National Institute of Diabetes and Digestive and Kidney Diseases, "Heartburn, Gastroesophageal Reflux (GER), and Gastroesophageal Reflux Disease (GERD)," April 30, 2012. http://digestive.niddk.nih.gov/ddiseases/pubs/gerd/index.aspx.
28. Eivind Ness-Jensen, Anna Lindam, Jesper Lagergren, and Kristian Hveem, "Changes in Prevalence, Incidence, and Spontaneous Loss of Gastro-Oesophageal Reflux Symptoms: A Prospective Population-Based Cohort Study, the HUNT Study," *Gut*, January 4, 2012. www.ntnu.edu/documents/139226/8932977/Gut-2011-Ness-Jensen-gutjnl-2011-300715.pdf.
29. Isaac J. Kassin, "First Person on Celiac Disease: How It Shaped My Life," Stewardship Report, November 22, 2012. http://stewardshipreport.com/celiac-disease-how-it-shaped-my-life.
30. Kassin, "First Person on Celiac Disease."
31. Kassin, "First Person on Celiac Disease."

Chapter 2: What Causes Digestive Disorders?

32. Barry J. Marshall, interviewed by Kathryn Schulz, "Stress Doesn't Cause Ulcers! Or, How to Win a Nobel Prize in One Easy Lesson: Barry Marshall on Being . . . Right," *The Wrong Stuff: What It Means to Make Mistakes* (blog), *Slate*, September 9, 2010. www.slate.com/blogs/thewrongstuff/2010/09/09/stress_doesn_t_cause_ulers_or_how_to_win_a_nobel_prize_in_one_easy_lesson_barry_marshall_on_being_right.html.
33. Marshall, interviewed by Schulz, "Stress Doesn't Cause Ulcers!"
34. National Institute of Diabetes and Digestive and Kidney Diseases, "*H. Pylori* and Peptic Ulcers," April 30, 2012. http://digestive.niddk.nih.gov/ddiseases/pubs/hpylori.
35. Quoted in Chris Iliades, "How Stress Affects Digestion," Everyday Health, 2013. www.everydayhealth.com/health-report/better-digestion/how-stress-affects-digestion.aspx.
36. National Institute of Diabetes and Digestive and Kidney Diseases, "Irritable Bowel Syndrome," July 2, 2012. http://digestive.niddk.nih.gov/ddiseases/pubs/ibs.
37. University of North Carolina at Chapel Hill School of Medicine, "What Causes Inflammatory Bowel Diseases (IBD)?," 2012. www.med.unc.edu/gi/ibd/what-causes-inflammatory-bowel-diseases-ibd.
38. University of North Carolina at Chapel Hill School of Medicine, "What Causes Inflammatory Bowel Diseases (IBD)?"
39. Institute of Diabetes and Digestive and Kidney Diseases, "Smoking and Your Digestive System," April 30, 2012. http://digestive.niddk.nih.gov/ddiseases/pubs/smoking.
40. Quoted in Salynn Boyles, "Antibiotics May Raise Bowel Disease Risk in Kids," WebMD, September 24, 2012. www.webmd.com/ibd-crohns-disease/news/20120924/antibiotics-bowel-disease-risk-kids.
41. National Institute of Diabetes and Digestive and Kidney Diseases, "Irritable Bowel Syndrome."

42. Quoted in Melinda Beck, "Clues to Gluten Sensitivity," *Wall Street Journal*, March 15, 2011. http://online.wsj.com/article/SB10001424052748704893604576200393522456636.html.

Chapter 3: What Are the Effects of Digestive Disorders?

43. Sophie Lee, "Guest Post: Sophie's Story with IBS," Healing Well, November 21, 2011. http://blog.healingwell.com/2011/11/guest-post-sophies-story-with-ibs.html.
44. Lee, "Guest Post: Sophie's Story with IBS."
45. Quoted in Watson, "6 Common Mistakes When You Have Crohn's Disease."
46. Quoted in Diana Rodriguez, "Living with Crohn's Disease: Janice's Story," Everyday Health, September 2, 2010. www.everydayhealth.com/crohns-disease/janices-story.aspx.
47. Quoted in Rodriguez, "Living with Crohn's Disease: Janice's Story."
48. Mayo Clinic, "GERD," April 13, 2012. www.mayoclinic.com/health/gerd/DS00967.
49. Kassin, "First Person on Celiac Disease."
50. Kassin, "First Person on Celiac Disease."
51. Jonathan LaPook, "Acid Reflux Doesn't Just Cause Heartburn," CBS News, October 1, 2009. www.cbsnews.com/2100-503823_162-5335730.html.
52. Jay W. Marks, "Peptic Ulcer Disease," MedicineNet, May 16, 2012. www.medicinenet.com/peptic_ulcer/article.htm.
53. Quoted in Ross Forman, "Buffalo Grove Boy Airlifted from Ship with Bleeding Ulcer," *Daily Herald* (suburban Chicago), April 2, 2011. www.dailyherald.com/article/20110401/news/704019883.
54. Quoted in Barbara Toman, "Celiac Disease: On the Rise," *Mayo Clinic Discovery's Edge*, July 2010. http://discoverysedge.mayo.edu/celiac-disease/index.cfm.
55. National Institutes of Health, "What People with Celiac Disease Need to Know About Osteoporosis," January 2012. www.niams.nih.gov/Health_Info/Bone/Osteoporosis/Conditions_Behaviors/celiac.asp.
56. Kassin, "First Person on Celiac Disease."

Chapter 4: How Are Digestive Disorders Treated?

57. John Sanford, "New Incision-Free Surgery Helps Tame Chronic Acid Reflux," Stanford University Medical Center, December 12, 2011. http://med.stanford.edu/ism/2011/december/reflux-1212.html.
58. J. Fernando del Rosario, "Gastroesophageal Reflux Disease (GERD)," Teens Health from Nemours, June 2011. http://kidshealth.org/teen/diseases_conditions/digestive/gerd.html.
59. National Institute of Diabetes and Digestive and Kidney Diseases, "*H. Pylori* and Peptic Ulcers."
60. Quoted in Amy Anderson, "A Gum to Cure Stomach Ulcers," *Daily Mail* (London), n.d. www.dailymail.co.uk/health/article-97549/A-gum-cure-stomach-ulcers.html.
61. Quoted in Anderson, "A Gum to Cure Stomach Ulcers."
62. Stephen R. Weinland, "Question: Why See a Psychologist When the Diagnosis Is IBS?," UNC Center for Functional GI & Motility Disorders, 2007. www.med.unc.edu/ibs/files/educational-gi-handouts/Seeing%20a%20Psychologist%20for%20IBS.pdf.
63. Weinland, "Question."
64. Weinland, "Question."
65. Quoted in Bill Hendrick, "Mindfulness Meditation May Cut IBS Symptoms," WebMD, May 10, 2011. www.webmd.com/ibs/news/20110510/mindfulness-meditation-may-cut-ibs-symptoms.
66. Quoted in Mikel Theobald, "Young and Living with Crohn's," Everyday Health, 2012. www.everydayhealth.com/crohns-disease/young-and-living-with-crohns.aspx.

List of Illustrations

Index

Note: Boldface page numbers indicate illustrations.

About the Author

Peggy J. Parks holds a bachelor of science degree from Aquinas College in Grand Rapids, Michigan, where she graduated magna cum laude. An author who has written more than a hundred educational books for children and young adults, Parks lives in Muskegon, Michigan, a town that she says inspires her writing because of its location on the shores of Lake Michigan.